Get Fit, Feel Great–Starting Today!

Top Personal Trainers From Around The Country Share Their Best Fitness Secrets

Rymor Publishing Group

DEDICATION

This book is dedicated to all of the incredible professionals and companies who took the time to submit content to this book. It has been a pleasure working with each of you, on the production of this book. The time you have all taken and the high quality content that you have all shared has truly gone above and beyond anything we could have ever expected when we first set out to publish this book. Thank you to everyone who made this possible.

CONTENTS

ACKNOWLEDGMENTS

We are deeply grateful to all the companies, who had a hand in making this incredible book possible. Our very special thanks goes out to:

Fit To You, LLC, McGannon Fitness & Nutrition, Unite Fitness, Attitude Dance & Fitness, LLC, Locke's Personal Fitness, Pure Fit Club, The Fitness Center at The Myerberg, Taylor Carpenter Personal Training, LLC, Saldare Body Therapy & Wellness Studio, Simple Fitness, Official Fitness Pro, Shuichi Take Fitness, Fitness4Life Training Center, Rundle Fit, and Fitness By Patty.

Facts and information are believed to be accurate at the time they were published in this book. All information provided is to be used for informational purposes only. Products and services described are only offered in jurisdictions where they may be legally offered. Information provided is not all-inclusive, and is limited to information that is made available. Such information should not be relied upon as all-inclusive or accurate.

You agree to hold Rymor Publishing Group, its owners, agents, and employees harmless from any and all liability for all claims for damages due to injuries, including attorney fees and costs, incurred by you or caused to third parties by you, arising out of the fitness and diet plans discussed in this book.

Testimonials, case studies, and examples within this book are unverified results that have been forwarded to us by the interviewees featured in this book, and may not reflect the typical reader's experience, may not apply to the average person, and are not intended to represent or guarantee that anyone will achieve the same or similar results. You should always perform due diligence and not take such results at face value. We are not responsible for any errors or omissions in typical results information supplied to us by third parties.

INTRODUCTION

If you've ever spent any amount of time strolling through the "Fitness & Nutrition" books section, at your local book store, you've probably noticed one thing: There sure are a lot of books on the subject of losing weight and eating healthy. While this large amount of information on the subject may seem like a good thing, it could also be the one thing that keeps you from taking action towards your personal fitness and nutrition goals.

As you're probably aware, the fitness and nutrition industry is a multi-billion dollar industry. There are thousands upon thousands of people who rely on you to buy the next fitness book, exercise gadget, or DVD that hits the store shelves or the late night TV airwaves. Unfortunately, in this profit-driven world known as the fitness and nutrition industry, one priority gets lost: Getting real results for the end-user. You see, if one of these multi-million dollar companies actually produced a gadget or DVD that enabled everyone to be in the best shape of their lives forever, you wouldn't need to buy their products anymore - and that's exactly what they don't want to happen!

So what does this mean for you? Should you just throw in the towel and give up on any and all information out there? Of course not. You do, however, need to be more selective in where you get your information from.

The goal of this book was to interview real personal trainers who really train clients each and every day of their professional lives. Inside this book, you're not going to find interviews with celebrity fitness trainers. As you probably realize, most celebrity fitness trainers do very little day-to-day fitness training, because it conflicts with their schedules of book signings, producing DVDs, and filming television commercials. It's sad to say, but many great personal trainers stop being great personal trainers the moment they get "discovered" by the "machine" that is the fitness and nutrition's marketing industry.

Consider this book to be the opposite of those glitzy, celebrity-endorsed books. When we produced this book, we set out to find real world experts and that's exactly what we got. Our biggest challenge was getting these personal trainers to break away from their busy schedules of training their clients, so that they could actually share their advice in this book. The trainers who have contributed to this book "walk the walk", and the content they've provided, in the following chapters, reflects their true knowledge and expertise. So, without further ado, we present to you, the real world expert interviews!

Chapter (1)

FIT TO YOU, LLC

"Answers provided by Ariana Gordon, Founder"

"Fit To You, LLC was created with a mission to aid individuals in improving their quality of life through physical wellness. While working as a personal trainer in various gyms, I was horrified to see the disregard for my clients from the management. To the management, my clients were dollar signs with various numbers listed afterward. I wanted to create a personal training company that puts humanity back into business. At Fit To You, LLC, we see our clients as people, not as numbers, and we keep the needs of our clients at the forefront of every decision we make. We remember the service component in the term "customer service" and try to exceed expectations in both client relations and quality of personal training services. Fit To You, LLC is a mobile company that specializes in one-on-one or group in-home, in-office, and web-based personal training as well as exercise program design."
~Ariana Gordon, Founder.

Q.) What should people look out for when hiring a personal trainer?

A.) Personal training is currently an unregulated industry. States do not offer any type of licensing program for personal trainers. This means that, unlike nurses, doctors, and lawyers, anyone can call themselves a personal trainer even if they know nothing about fitness. Consequently, there are a lot of terrible trainers. The first thing people should look for when hiring a personal trainer is a NCCA accredited personal training certification. As far as certifications go, we have what is referred to as the "top 4". If you are hiring a personal trainer, they should have a certification from one of the "top 4", which includes: American Council on Exercise, National Academy of Sports Medicine, National Strength and Conditioning Association, American College of Sports

Medicine. While talking to prospective trainers, do not be afraid to ask who they are certified through and pick their brain a bit. If the trainer does not seem to know what they are talking about, run. Another component to take into consideration when hiring a personal trainer is personality. If a person does not like their personal trainer, they are unlikely to attend sessions on a regular basis and they are unlikely to continue training until they reach their goal. If you want to accomplish whatever you are hiring the personal trainer for, you have to like them.

Q.) If someone has a friend who is in good shape, who is willing to give them exercise advice, why is it still a good idea to hire a personal trainer?

A.) A lot of people think they know how to exercise, but really do not. Just because a friend looks like they are in good shape does not mean they know what they are doing. Training with someone who is not a professional sets you up for injury and can be very damaging in the long run.

Q.) Is it true that people should take periods of time off from working out? If so, how long should these "workout vacations" last and how frequently should they occur?

A.) Yes and no. Over-training is a very real problem, but I do not advocate stopping exercise completely. I prevent my clients from over-training by doing exercises with weights that are much lighter than they are used to. This way the muscles are not completely sedentary, they are still doing the same motions, but they are not being overloaded. These "rest days" can be one session or a full week depending on the person and how heavy their normal weights are. I include these "rest days" approximately every 6 weeks.

Q.) What are some tips to help people stick with an exercise program and not quit?

A.) I am a big fan of behavioral modification techniques. Usually, internal desire and intended commitment are not enough to motivate a person. If a person adds an external reward for healthy habits, they are much more likely to succeed in their endeavor. For example, I have a client who has been struggling to control her emotional eating at night. When I discussed some sort of prize program with her, she stated that the ability to save money is a big motivator for her. The prize program that she created for herself is to put a quarter in a savings jar every night that she does not snack. For myself, I pick out items that I really want to buy and put in place requirements to buy them. I bought myself a new guitar last month as a reward for hitting one of my goals – this month, it was a pair of shoes. If you want something badly enough, you will do whatever it takes to get it.

Q.) What is a "drop set"?

A.) A drop set is a method of training in which you start off with heavier weights on the first set and reduce the amount of weight for each subsequent set. This is particularly popular among bodybuilders because it allows the person to push their body to failure multiple times. It is not the safest method of weight training for the general population and should be used sparingly.

Q.) If someone likes to listen to music, on a personal music player with headphones, when they workout, is this considered rude by most personal trainers?

A.) Yes, listening to music through headphones while working with a trainer is considered rude. If the person has in only one of the earbuds, this would be slightly more acceptable. When clients listen to music through headphones while working with a trainer, the verbal cues and corrections that the trainer gives become less effective and it is typically more difficult to get the client's attention when you need it. This happens for two reasons: first, the client's hearing capabilities are reduced so they are less likely to hear the trainer and second, the trainer does not know how much the client can hear and will tend to give the client fewer corrections.

Q.) Which types of people can benefit the most from a personal trainer?

A.) In my opinion, everyone can benefit from a personal trainer because very few people know how to exercise safely and correctly. There are some people, however, that should not attempt any form of exercise without a personal trainer. These would be people with injuries (new or old), people who are severely deconditioned, and people who have no experience with strength training.

Q.) What are "boot camps" and why are they so popular?

A.) Boot camps are group classes with a mix of strength training and cardio exercises designed to push participants to their physical maximum. Boot camps are extremely popular because they include a social component and, afterward, people feel like they have accomplished more than they thought they could. Boot camps are what you would think of when you are looking for military-style training.

Q.) How can people overcome junk food cravings?

A.) With most foods, you can find a healthier alternative. Chocolate milk is a great way to combat a craving for sweets. Kale chips could give you the crunch and saltiness of potato chips. I always tell my clients to have everything in moderation, though. I do not want my clients to try to cut out junk food altogether, because it would result in binge eating the junk food at some point. It is alright to have the food that you are craving, just be careful about how much of it you will allow yourself to eat.

Q.) Do most personal trainers yell at people, like drill sergeants, to keep them motivated? What if someone wants to hire a personal trainer without being screamed at?

A.) Not at all! I've actually never met a personal trainer who yelled at their clients like a drill sergeant. Every personal trainer has their own unique style and their own unique personality. It is important that you find a personal trainer with a personality and style that fits yours. Finding a personal trainer that does not scream at you will not be difficult.

Q.) How does someone know if they're "over-training"?

A.) The biggest indication of over-training is fatigue. Mentally and physically, the person will slow down and be very low on energy. If someone is struggling to finish a set of an exercise with the same weights and reps they have used previously, consider if they have any new stresses in their life. If the person is sleeping normally, is otherwise in good health, and has eaten well that day, there is a good chance that their difficulty finishing the set is caused by over-training.

Q.) How will a trainer know what program is right for their client?

A.) During the first few sessions, trainers learn their clients' bodies. We base our programs on what muscle compensations need to be corrected, along with the clients' goals. Personal training is an art – not all paintings look the same, but a good painter can turn every one of their works of art into a masterpiece.

Q.) Is it typically acceptable for people to bring their children to a personal training session?

A.) Typically no, but it depends on the situation. If the children are well behaved, most trainers will not have a problem with the children being present during the session. I have a client who brings her son with her and he sits against the wall playing on his PSP, so it is not a problem. As long as the children don't hinder the client's performance during our session, I don't care if they are there.

Q.) How much sleep should people get when they exercise regularly?

A.) Everyone's body is unique, so there is no one number of hours that every person should get. Some people only need six hours of sleep and others need twelve. I encourage my clients to listen to their body and maintain a sensitivity to its signals. The one piece of advice regarding sleep that I do give to every client is to wake up at the end of a 90 minute interval. Sleep cycles run in 90 minute intervals and you will feel much less rested if you wake up in the middle of a sleep cycle than if you get slightly less sleep and wake up at the end of a sleep cycle. So, instead of getting 8 hours of sleep per night, go for 7.5 or 9. You will feel the difference.

Thank you Ariana...

If you would like to learn more about Fit To You, LLC, their information will follow.

Ariana Gordon, Founder
www.FitToYouLLC.com
443.970.0934
www.facebook.com/FitToYouPersonalTraining
www.twitter.com/FitToYouLLC

Chapter (2)

MCGANNON FITNESS & NUTRITION

"Answers provided by Wendy McGannon, Owner"

McGannon Fitness & Nutrition was founded in 2008 by Wendy McGannon. She became a trainer to address her own chronic neck, shoulder and back pain which resulted from sitting at a desk all day long. She became frustrated with the lack of change that occurred regardless of multiple modes of body work (massage, acupuncture, chiropractic, physical therapy). She learned which muscles needed to be strengthened, which needed to be stretched (and how) and she added regular strength training, cardio, and stretching to the body work that she had been doing. The end result was no more chronic pain!

Approximately 85% of the clients we train are women between the ages of 40 – 60's. Most of them have desk jobs and suffer from some sort of pain issue. Our goal is to help them to decrease or eliminate their pain, increase their core strength, balance and stability, and increase their overall strength and ability to do more of the things they could not do previously. Almost all of them succeed!

"I love being a personal trainer and nutrition coach because I get to work with great people who are trying to improve the quality of their lives. I believe that everyone can reach their health and fitness goals but many people need help getting started. Accurate information and accountability provide the groundwork to create healthier eating and exercise habits in a balanced way that can be maintained over time." ~ Wendy McGannon

Q.) What are the must-have items that someone should bring with them to a personal training session?

A.) Must-have items to bring to a personal training session include water, comfortable clothing that will allow free movement of the body, and supportive foot wear. Not essential but certainly helpful would also include sports bras for women, heart-rate monitors, and a willingness to work hard. Depending on the level of impact and intensity the participant will be engaging in, the sports bra and the HR monitor may be moved into the essential category, especially for the elite or more athletic clients.

Q.) What are some of the most common myths about losing weight?

A.) Many people believe if they skip meals, they will lose weight. Unfortunately, this habit often has the reverse effect than intended. When people skip meals, they are slowing their metabolism down somewhat and burning calories at a reduced rate than if they had eaten a healthy, reasonable meal. Additionally, when we wait too long between meals to eat, we are often more hungry and prone to making worse food choices and/or overeating.

Another myth is that all carbs are bad. Carbohydrates are contained within all fruits and vegetables. When people go on a diet that eliminates all carbs, they are losing all of the essential vitamins, minerals, and nutrients contained within the lower calories fruit and vegetable food groups. While it is certainly true that many people eat way too many unhealthy, processed carbohydrates, there are many good carbs that are essential for life. Whole grains, in moderation, are a very important part of a healthy diet.

A third myth that many people seem to get stuck on is that they have to give up all the unhealthy foods they love in order to lose weight. This myth is probably the most harmful and one that leads to "diet" failure rates most frequently.

If we remember that a pound of fat is equal to 3,500 calories, we will need to restrict daily caloric intake by 500 calories in order to lose one pound of fat per week, assuming we are not exercising. Conversely, we can burn an additional 500 calories per day to lose the same pound per week or combine the calorie restriction with the extra calorie burn to lose 2 pounds per week.

We do not need to give up all the foods we love when trying to lose weight. What we do need to do is eat healthier foods more often, eat few calories over the course of the day, and still eat several small meals that will help to maintain our blood sugar levels and not leave us feeling deprived or starving. Sometimes an occasional fast food meal or donut is what we want and need to give ourselves to ultimately stay on track in the long run. Small changes that we accumulate over time result in lifestyle changes that we can maintain.

Q.) Other than losing weight and gaining muscle, what are some of the other benefits of getting in shape?

A.) One of the main benefits of getting in shape is the ability to maintain functionality as we age, especially for clients over 40. Being able to engage in activities of daily living without back, neck, shoulder, and sciatica pain is a huge benefit, not to mention the increases in balance, stability, and stamina.

Other benefits include:

- lower blood pressure
- lower overall cholesterol levels (bad – LDL decreases and good – HDL increases)
- lower risk of diabetes
- increased metabolism – ability to burn more calories on an ongoing basis
- increased cardio respiratory efficiency and endurance
- increased bone mass (decreased risk of osteoporosis)
- decreased levels of stress

- better posture and self esteem

Q.) What can people do if they "plateau" and stop seeing results from their workout routine?

A.) They need to change their workout routine. Our bodies will adapt to whatever exercises we do on a regular basis. The more variable our workouts, the less chance our bodies have of adapting and reaching a plateau. Some clients feel more comfortable with a regular routine and don't want to be varying their exercises. The way around the plateau for these clients is to have them shift the number or repetitions, the amount of weight, and/or the number of sets they are completing. These changes can be made every 4 – 6 weeks to help clients to see ongoing improvements.

Q.) Is it a bad idea to eat right after working out? Why or why not?

A.) It is a bad idea NOT to eat after a workout. Eating post-workout is essential to refuel the body and rebuild muscles, especially after hard workouts. Protein is crucial for muscle growth and carbohydrates (which are most easily metabolized after workouts) are helpful to replenish the body's glycogen (or fuel) stores that help keep us going. A healthy balance of lean protein, whole grain carbohydrates, and plenty of water are really important post workout.

Q.) What should someone do if they get muscle cramps during a workout? Should they work through it or do something else?

A.) A muscle cramp is a sign from the body that something is wrong and it should not be ignored and "worked through". Muscle cramps can be caused by lack of hydration, especially in conjunction with muscle contraction. People should drink water, massage the affected area, and stretch the cramping muscle before continuing to work out. Foam rolling can be a very effective tool to help with muscle tightness. If the muscle continues to cramp, give it a rest and continue to massage and stretch it while properly hydrating the whole body (minimum of 8 – 12 eight ounce glasses of water per day).

Q.) How can someone tell if their personal trainer's certification is legitimate?

A.) Ask them for a copy of the certification which will have the certifying agency name and certification number on it. If they do not produce the copy, ask them for the above information and go online to the agency to look the person up. Trainers are required to keep their certifications up to date by engaging in ongoing professional development. If someone has not done so, this will be evident online (i.e, the certifying agency will list the trainer's certification as expired).

Q.) Is there any true benefit to warming up, cooling down, or stretching before or after exercising? If there is, why are these things important?

A.) Absolutely, and there is also importance to doing specific types of warming up, cooling, down, and stretching. Dynamic warm up (moving stretches) are essential to get the muscles ready to contract, especially for more intense workouts. If we don't warm up our muscles, we increase the risk of harming ourselves by straining or pulling muscles. The dynamic warm up allows our muscles to stretch and get ready to contract in a way that helps keep the body safe. When we are done with our workout (e.g. we have finished contracting or shortening our muscles) it's really important to engage in static (or holding) stretches to bring the muscles back to their elongated state. It is also very important to hold post workout stretches for 20 – 30 seconds each in order to help the muscles to release, reduce the amount of metabolic waste left in the muscles, and reduce the level of soreness we will feel after our workouts.

Q.) Why is it important for people to work on improving their balance and how can they do this?

A.) Balance is an essential skill that people need to have to move through the world safely. This skill becomes increasingly important as people age. Without exercise, bones become more brittle and muscles become weaker. If a person loses balance and falls, their likelihood of breaking bones increases exponentially as they get older.

Balance is improved by helping people to strengthen their core muscles and understand how to use their core in all activities of living, not just while they are working out. Besides strengthening the core muscles, it is essential to strengthen all of the larger and smaller muscles throughout the leg, butt, and ankles. Bosu balance trainers are an excellent tool to help with this but are somewhat expensive (approximately $100). Standing on one leg is a free way to work on increasing stabilizing muscles throughout the leg and ankle. Adding heel raises will also help to strengthen the ankles. Core strength is more complicated and a trainer is essential to helping ensure that people are strengthening in ways that are not going to hurt their backs, necks, or otherwise cause pain or injury to themselves.

Q.) What is the correct way to breathe when working out?

A.) It is typically recommended that a person breath in during the easier part of the exercise (the "down" movement of the push up for example) and breath out during the exertion, or hard part of the exercise (e.g., pushing away from the floor during the push up). Many people benefit from this advice, especially during intense exertions, however; some clients who struggle with proper form during exercises tend to become overwhelmed when they try to remember how to breathe during an exercise. It just becomes one more thing they have to think about. A trainer needs to asses each client's individual skills and needs before focusing on breathing techniques with them.

Q.) If a particular exercise hurts, is that normal?

A.) It depends on where the "hurt" is felt and how intense it is. Minor discomfort in a muscle is normal because we are asking our muscles to contract, or shorten, often with additional weight pulling or pushing on the muscle. The weaker our muscles and the more weight we are using, the more discomfort we are likely to feel. If there is intense pain in a muscle or if there is any pain in a joint, this is not normal and the exercise should be stopped immediately. If a person is working with a trainer, they need to communicate very clearly with the trainer about any joint pain or severe muscle pain to ensure that the trainer can modify or change the exercise to protect the client. It is the trainer's job to push clients a little bit beyond their comfort zone and it is the client's job to clearly communicate about levels of discomfort to maintain safety.

Q.) What is "core strength"?

A.) Our "core" refers to all of the muscles in our abdominal area as well as several of the muscles in our back, essentially, the muscles throughout our trunk region. When we talk about core strength, we are referring to the body's ability to contract these muscles. Core strength is really important because our core muscles connect all of the movements of our lower and upper body and help us to maintain our balance as we move through the various activities of our lives.

Many people refer to core strength in terms of abdominal strength, which is slightly inaccurate but fine for the purposes of understanding its importance. The stronger our abdominal muscles are and the more we learn how to use them, the more we are able to protect our back muscles. Many people pull muscles in their backs when lifting heavy objects because they are not effectively using their core (in conjunction with their quadriceps – leg muscles, and biceps – arm muscles) or their core is simply not strong enough to help with the movement and the muscles in the back try to help. Unfortunately our back muscles were not designed for heavy lifting and often become strained or pulled during these movements.

Another way core strength helps us to protect our backs is by helping us to improve our posture. When we pull our belly button toward our spine, our shoulders automatically move back, opening up our chest. When we contract our core (or abdominal) muscles to maintain this position we stop pulling on the muscles of our back and neck because we are sitting up straight with our necks in line with our spines, rather than slumping over.

Core strength is key to everything we do while exercising and while engaging in activities of daily living safely. Many people overdue the core training and/or engage in exercises improperly which results in injury to their backs. A trainer can be very helpful in designing a safe core strengthening program.

Thank you Wendy...

If you would like to learn more about, McGannon Fitness & Nutrition, their information will follow.

McGannon Fitness & Nutrition is located at 15 College Highway, Suite G1 in Southampton, Massachusetts

Please visit us online at: www.mcgannonfitness.com

Other contact information:
mcgannonfitness@gmail.com
(413) 297-2590

Chapter (3)

UNITE FITNESS

"Answers provided by Juliet Burgh, NASM, CHC"

"Unite Fitness was born from our Heart.Muscle.Mind [HMM] philosophy, which is an integrated view and training program that unites all the elements necessary for a healthy, active lifestyle that results in a lean muscular body. HMM is an evolving approach that is rooted in essential and proven principles of using cardiovascular training (the heart), strength training (the muscle) and yoga (the mind). Years of study and practice have enabled us to unite these elements of fitness into one smart, balanced, kick ass program. Unite has also developed it's signature nutrition program and eating philosophy to help people achieve their goals even faster." ~Juliet Burgh

Q.) If someone eats very healthy, and they have an active lifestyle, do they still need to work out? Why or why not?

A.) It depends on what kind of active lifestyle they are leading. I think it is important to get your heart rate elevated to increase blood and oxygen to the body, strengthen the cardiovascular system and stimulate the brain to produce "feel good" chemicals. So if their activity is just a leisurely walk around the park, I would say they would benefit from a more intense activity like hiking or biking.

Q.) Do minors typically need to get the permission of an adult or guardian, if they want to work with a personal trainer? If so, how does this work?

A.) Yes, minors do need permission to work with a trainer. It is important that we obtain consent when working with someone who does not have a fully developed body. Strength training can change body composition and although this can be a positive thing, if done improperly there can be consequences. An example would be gymnasts bodies who over grow their muscles from a young age and it can impact their adult growth patterns and look of the body. The way we obtain consent is by discussing with the guardian the goal of the minor and what we intend to do as we work with them. We have them sign a consent form for legality.

Q.) Why do some people lift heavy weights while other people lift lighter amounts of weights?

A.) There are several reasons people lift heavy weights vs. light weights. A lot of it is what they have heard from someone. Different trainers have a certain perspective, philosophy and personal taste that can be transferred to their clients. There is science that backs resistance training as being a great way to build healthy muscle tissue and build bone density, however resistance training can come in many forms, i.e.: using light weights, using your body weight or using heavy weights. There are also some negative associations that come with lifting heavy weights that can skew a person's opinion. You often look at bulky body builders and assume that heavy weights will give you that particular body. From experience and working with clients, I have many lean and toned females who lift very heavy and do not grow larger muscles. If anything, it burns more calories when lifting heavy, because you can put more load on your body and make your strength training more challenging.

Q.) Do personal trainers normally work with clients who are only free on weekends or during off-hours? What's typical in terms of when personal trainers are available?

A.) Most full time personal trainers adhere to client's schedules, whether that be early morning before work clients (5am-8am), afternoon lunch clients (12-3pm) or after work evening clients (4:00-8pm) and weekends as well. If you are a part-time personal trainer you would work with clients before work, after work and on weekends only.

Q.) If someone has back problems, or other physical limitations, how can they lift weights safely, without getting hurt?

A.) We can use more stabilized exercises with a client like this. Machines and seated exercises can be helpful for clients who need a lot of support, as well as not pushing the client to go beyond their limitations. Using proper weights and form is key.

Q.) What is the typical way to pay a personal trainer? Weekly? Monthly? At each session?

A.) Personal trainers who work for a company get paid bi-weekly or weekly for the amount of sessions that that accumulated in that time. Clients purchase packages of sessions (10, 25, 40) up front, and the trainer gets paid as sessions are completed. If you work for yourself you might have a client pay you before or after each individual session or at the end of the week. It is up to the trainer if they are independent.

Q.) When is a spotter needed for exercises?

A.) When lifting extremely heavy weights or when working with a client who is a beginner and needs work on getting correct form down. A trainer might guide them the whole way.

Q.) How does someone tone up in specific "problem areas"?

A.) There is no such thing as spot reduction. For example, you can't chew gum all day expecting your cheeks to thin out. We have to focus on the whole body to get overall fat reduction and wherever the body wants to shed fat first it will. You can however work a problem area that is not for vanity. If you have weak hamstrings you can perform specific exercises that will strengthen them over time.

Q.) Is it true that too much cardio can be unhealthy?

A.) Yes, too much cardio can increase cortisol levels and cause the body to store body fat. It also can cause digestive issues, hormonal issues and over-exercise syndrome due to too much stress on the body and lack of recovery time.

Q.) What are the benefits of hiring a personal trainer over just buying some DVDs that feature personal trainers?

A.) Personal trainers can not only support you and motivate you they can really help you with the proper form and ways of doing the exercise. Watching a DVD doesn't have the same effect. You also get to know your personal trainer and they get to know you. Over time he or she will find out what the right things to say to you are that can be stimulating and helpful. A DVD will never know you and the name of your dog. A personal relationship can help you to look forward to your workouts and stick to a program.

Q.) Is it a good idea to walk or run with weights? Will this produce results more quickly?

A.) It's not a bad idea. Using weights while you walk or run can get your heart rate up faster and cause your upper body muscles to work harder than they would if you didn't use weights. You can gain fast results from a variety of different workouts on your body, so if you enjoy the walking or running with weights then go ahead and do it. I wouldn't walk or run with weight every day, because it can put extra stress on the joints, but it is something you can incorporate into your routine a few times a week.

Q.) How soon, after someone starts a diet and exercise program, should they start to see results, to know if their diet and exercise program is working?

A.) You should feel results within 1 week if you are changing your diet properly. You can judge this by 1-2 lbs lost on the scale or an overall feeling of having more energy and feeling lighter. Exercise can take 2-4 weeks to really feel the difference. Being sore after a workout can make you feel like it's working, but isn't a great judge of whether or not it is.

Q.) What are some of the most common misconceptions that people have about hiring a personal trainer?

- That personal trainers will act like a drill sergeant and make people do things that they don't necessarily want to do.
- That personal trainers are super humans and can't understand regular peoples upsets about body and diet. We are regular people who have to work hard at this just like you.
- That hiring a trainer will be like a magic pill and within a short amount of time they will have the body of their dreams.
- Clients think they can come in 1-2x per week and get results. It takes at least 3-6 days per week to get vanity results.

Q.) What are some of the most common myths about nutrition?

- Carbs are bad
- Fat is bad
- Eating less and exercising more is the way to lose weight
- Eat as many fruits and vegetables as you want and you won't gain weight
- Health food tastes bad
- That you have to be 100% on a diet all the time. (all or nothing mentality)
- Fad diets work long term
- More protein is better for you

Thank you Juliet...

If you would like to learn more about Unite Fitness, their information will follow.

www.unitefitness.com
juliet@unitefitness.com

Juliet Burgh, NASM, CHC
Unite Fitness
Partner/Nutrition Director
Telephone: (845) 399-3055
Website: unitefitness.com

Chapter (4)

ATTITUDE DANCE AND FITNESS, LLC

"Answers provided by Robyn DiNatale, CPT"

"Attitude Dance and Fitness, LLC was founded in 2006 as primarily a children's dance studio. Having been in the fitness industry most of my life, and responding to the needs of women in the area of not being able to find an all adult women's dance class, I decided to combine both fitness and dance with a fun alternative to a traditional Ballet class. Ballet Boot Camp/Ballet Fitness is a total body workout that incorporates core work, balance and stabilization for the enhancement of fat burning even well after your workout is done! A variety of different classes are taught under "Ballet Fitness" which makes each and every single class unique no matter how many classes per week you participate in. Attitude Dance and Fitness is a low-key, comfortable, nurturing studio where every "body" feels welcome! Located in the beautiful shoreline town of Branford, Ct."   *~Robyn DiNatale*

Q.) What should a personal trainer take into consideration when working with each individual client?

A.) The answer is right in the question. "Individual." While there are certain protocols that should always be followed, each client has their own special needs, goals etc...And therefore must be approached as an individual and not necessarily by the book.

Q.) If someone isn't sore after a workout, does that mean they didn't work out hard enough?

A.) Not always. It depends on what type of workout it was and/or did the person do the same or similar workout recently. Was there (hopefully) a significant warm-up, cool-down, stretching? All can be factors effecting the level of soreness and post workout.

Q.)The new fad seems to be "buying organic". Is there any validity to eating organic food over non-organic food? What are the benefits and/or things to be aware of?

A.) I try to educate my clients to eat sensibly without extreme. Organic food tends to be much more expensive and one needs to be aware that "organic" doesn't automatically translate to healthy or low fat. If pesticides are a concern for you then by all means buy organic but be sure to look for certified organic products USDA on the label.

Q.) Should people wait until they're not sore from their previous workout to start working out again?

A.) There should be rest days between heavy, intense training. Training the same body parts successively is not a good idea as the rest is what allows the muscles to grow but one should also keep in mind that everyone experiences soreness differently. It also depends on the level of soreness and where it is located.

Q.) If someone reaches their fitness goals, should they still continue to work with a personal trainer?

A.) This is a decision that only the client and the Personal Trainer can decide and there are so many variables that can come into play. For example, does this client have the motivation to sustain these goals that were reached? Financial situation? As a Personal Trainer, I try to arm my clients with the tools and skills they will need to go out and hopefully make this a way of life...on their own. But they are always welcome to continue if that's what they truly need.

Q.) When people first start exercising, why do they sometimes gain weight initially?

A.) Sometimes people can experience an increase in lean muscle tissue which is what we're striving for before the weight actually starts coming off. Muscle weighs more than fat. As a new exerciser your body needs time to adjust to the new demands being placed on it.

Q.) If someone has a heart condition, can they still work out?

A.) They would need their doctor's consent and it would depend on the exact condition but for many heart patients it is a good idea to exercise to help strengthen their heart muscle.

Q.) If someone has a job where they don't move around a lot, what can they do to increase their activity during the day, when they're not working out?

A.) Take short breaks where they can stretch. Do isometric movements at their desks which can be done with no one else noticing. Take a short walk on your lunch break. If you have an excuse to go to a different part of the building use the stairs instead of the elevator. It all adds up.

Q.) Is it safe for pregnant women to work out?

A.) Usually if they were already routinely working out prior and their doctors agree that they're having a normal pregnancy. As the pregnancy progresses, adjustments will need to be made.

Q.) If someone prefers to work out without a personal trainer, can a trainer still help them get started?

A.) How would this work? I offer a one session option where I can give them advice and guidance and gyms /health clubs usually, also, do the same helping to the get the client oriented.

Q.) Can someone use a personal trainer to help them rehabilitate from a sports injury? How would this be handled?

A.) Absolutely, but I would hope the trainer would hold a special cert for sports rehab. When it comes to nutrition, it seems that few experts can agree on what is a healthy diet and what is not. How can people know which advice to take, with all of the contradictory information out there? So much of it is common sense and trial and error. In general, a healthy diet is a diet consisting of a proper balance of protein, carbs, fruits and vegetables. As for alcohol, junk food etc... The old rule everything in moderation is key.

Q.) If a personal trainer is always showing up late, should the client still be expected to pay for the full session? What's the customary way to deal with a situation like this?

A.) Being a Personal Trainer, I've only been on the opposite end of this in which case I'll still give the client who's late the "remainder" of their session. If they have a legitimate excuse and I don't have another appointment directly after, I'll give them the whole session. If I were the client I'd have to question the professionalism of this trainer who is always running late?

Q.) Is it a good idea to eat any specific foods immediately before or after exercising?

A.) Before exercise, it's a good idea to have a light snack, like a carb (fruit, peanut butter crackers) especially if it's been a long time since you've last eaten so as to not get light headed. Generally speaking, it's usually a good idea to replenish your body after your workout with the nutrients you've used up.

Thank you Robyn...

If you would like to learn more about, Attitude Dance and Fitness, LLC, their information will follow.

Attitude Dance and Fitness (Ballet Fitness and Personal Training)
116 N Main St Branford, Ct 06405
203-641-1617
www.attitudedanceandfitness.com
robyn@attitudedanceandfitness.com

Thanks!
Robyn DiNatale, CPT
203-641-1617
http://attitudedanceandfitness.com

Rymor Publishing Group

This page intentionally left blank

Chapter (5)

LOCKE'S PERSONAL FITNESS

"Answers provided by Sherry J. Locke,
ACSM Certified Personal Trainer"

"Locke's Personal Fitness, was established in August of 1994 in Pittsburgh, Pennsylvania. Since then, we've opened up a personal training studio in April of 2001, relocated to expand in April of 2006, expanded again in 2010 and trained hundreds of people ranging in ages from children to seniors. Most people are looking to improve their overall health, some have specific goals, many want to lose weight, some are looking for sport-specific training, and then there are those who just finished physical therapy and are referred to us for continued supervised exercise.

All of our trainers either hold a degree in Exercise Science and/or hold one of the following certifications: ACSM (American College of Sports Medicine), ACE (American Council on Exercise) or NSCA (National Strength and Conditioning Association).

Our philosophy on nutrition is to teach our clients how to eat for better health and optimal weight. We do not sell or suggest supplements. We work with doctors and dietitians to get reliable and current information.

Some of our clients work with us for several weeks, some we've maintained since we opened the studio in 2001. We have people return after years of being on their own to get back on track. Our prices are discounted for frequency to encourage consistent exercise and to keep their eating habits on track. Many people just need (and want) to be held accountable for their behaviors. They tend to eat better on the days they know they are working out with us!

We train our clients mainly in our studio in Bethel Park, Pennsylvania (a suburb of Pittsburgh), but we still travel to work with clients in their homes if that's what makes them more comfortable." ~Sherry Locke

Q.) What are some of the biggest mistakes that people make when they start an exercise program?

1. They think that the more out of shape they are the more difficult the workout needs to be or the more severely they need to restrict their calorie intake.

2. They attempt to "spot reduce" by working the undesirable body part to death. Spot reduction is not possible without surgical intervention!

3. They get hypnotized by infomercials so they waste money on diets and unnecessary exercise equipment

Q.) How does someone know how hard to push themselves when they're working out?

A.) For beginner exercises, they need to start off with one set of each exercise and bring themselves to fatigue. Then, see how they feel (recover) in the next 24-48 hours. If they experience muscle stiffness to the point that they are limping or can't function normally, they've over-done it and know to scale back the resistance or repetitions on the next workout. If they felt nothing, then they can add another set (up to 3 sets). What everyone needs to remember is that they want to gradually increase strength and flexibility over time – not break it down. This is the difference between working with a trainer who knows what they are doing and working with a "gymrat" or the trainer with the online certification.

Q.) If someone just recently had surgery, can they lift weights or workout?

A.) Before someone begins or resumes a weight training program after surgery, they should ask their physician. That would go for C-sections too.

Q.) What should be taken into consideration in these situations?

A.) Someone who had been exercising regularly will most likely recover from a surgery or an injury faster than a sedentary person, not just from a fitness standpoint but from the severity of the surgery. If someone at a normal, healthy weight has surgery, there is less tissue to cut through and therefore less sutures or stitches hence the faster recovery and return to activities. These people will be back in action faster than someone who was overweight and had more tissue damage during the surgery equaling more sutures, stitches, pain and possibly complications.

Q.) Is it possible to lose fat and gain muscle at the same time?

A.) Yes, it is possible to lost fat and gain muscle at the same time. This is why we take girth measurements and skin fold measurements. The scale does not always reflect one's progress with respect to fat loss.

Q.) If so, how can this be done effectively?

A.) Changing one's diet is the most effective way to lose weight along with cardiovascular exercise to burn calories. When muscles begin to hypertrophy (grow), they become harder as well. Most people know that muscle is denser than body fat, but they don't know that muscle is metabolically active tissue. The more muscle a person has, the more calories they'll burn doing anything from sleeping to running.

Q.) If someone has been a "yo-yo dieter" their entire lives, how can a personal trainer help people like this?

A.) A knowledgeable personal trainer can explain to the dieter why the yo-yo method failed them. If someone is overweight, their first instinct is to eat less. I've been a personal trainer since 1994 and have worked with many overweight clients and consulted with no less than four dietitians. Once my client completed a nutritional analysis for the dietitian, the results would show that the client was NOT EATING ENOUGH. The reason for their repeated weight gain is most likely due to a slower metabolism. Metabolism can slow down for several reasons. Reason #1 is their age. A person's metabolism decreases approximately 2% per decade over the age of 30. Reason #2 is inactivity. Adults just don't make the time to play or exercise. Reason #3 is they try to combat the weight gain by eating less – and slowing their metabolism even more. Once they are tired of starving themselves, and they've slowed their metabolism even more by inadequate calorie intake, they gain weight when they increase their calories to their pre-diet level. A fourth and fifth reason for a slowing metabolism could also be due to an undiagnosed medical condition such as hypothyroid disease or even a medication that causes weight gain unbeknownst to the patient.

Q.) What is the difference between a "high impact" and a "low impact" workout?

A.) A high-impact workout is a workout that involves both feet being off the floor at the same time – even if it's just for a fraction of a second. Some examples of a high-impact exercise would be running, jumping jacks and plyometrics. Low -impact workouts will always have one foot in contact with the floor. Examples of this would be using an elliptical trainer where both feet remain in contact with the pedals at all times or walking because one foot is always on the ground. I think it's easy for people confuse "high and low *impact*" with "high and low *intensity*".

Q.) How much of a say should the client have in determining which exercises they do?

A.) Personally, I welcome feedback from my clients regarding their exercises. Not just because I need to listen to them when they tell me something is too difficult or the exercise is painful, but to help them adhere to their program. If I make a client do exercises they absolutely dread doing, there is a strong possibility they could be a frequent canceller or just quit. A good trainer will know many exercises for each muscle group. Sometimes, I'll even do a "client's choice" workout where I tell them what body part we are about to work and give them a choice of two or three exercises we can do for that muscle group. It also gives them a little control back during their workout too. I know sometimes I'm just not in the mood to do squats, so I'll do the leg press. Why shouldn't they have the same freedom of choice (sometimes)?

Q.) Why do certain "non-fat" foods still make people gain weight?

A.) Probably because they don't realize that when they take the fat out of a food, they usually load it up with sugar. Then there are the folks who eat more than they would if the food had fat in it in the first place.

Q.) Is it true that some exercises produce results faster than others?

A.) Sure, but it also depends on the effort and accuracy of the exercise being performed.

Q.) If so, which exercises provide the best and worst "returns on investment"?

A.) As far as investment of time, I tell people to avoid "tic toc" exercises for the waistline. At most, for their effort, they'll thicken the waist which is most likely not the intended goal. As far as investment of dollars, stay away from ab gadgets. They take up too much space, one size does not fit all (different torso lengths effect some of these apparatuses) and anyone purchasing an abdominal gadget is most likely doing so with the hopes of whittling away their midsection (spot reducing) which, as I mentioned earlier, is not possible without surgical intervention. Properly-executed ab curls and oblique exercises done on the floor, stability ball or BOSU with or without external resistance are the way to go.

Q.) How should someone determine how many grams of protein and carbs they should be eating each day?

A.) Do what I do and ask the most knowledgeable person on the subject – a dietitian (not to be confused with a nutritionist). My dietitian has given me a formula to use on the average client for protein. When it comes to carbs, I have them follow the guidelines set by the American Diabetes Association. If I have a client with low blood sugar, then they should consult with a dietitian for special guidelines. Most of my clients do well following the advice of the American Diabetes Association.

Q.) Is it a good idea for someone to work out if they have a cold?

A.) The guideline for exercising while sick is that it's okay to work out if the illness is from the neck up, but any lower (or fever) it should be avoided. The body uses vitamins and minerals consumed through food for growth, maintenance and repair of cells. If the exerciser is sick, they should let their body use all of its resources to fight the illness. Although, they can work out and use those resources to replenish what was lost during exercise. In this case, the most effective exercise would be that of using their common sense.

Q.) Is it better to perform cardio before or after lifting weights or should cardio be done on a completely different day?

A.) There are arguments for either, but the fact is, there is no solid scientific proof of either being the correct method. It's more of a preference. Some argue that cardio first is a nice long warm-up before the strength training. Then others argue that they need the majority of their energy to get through the strength training. The American College of Sports Medicine suggests cardiovascular training be done for an hour on most days of the week. When planning to do a strength training program for all of the muscle groups, that will take another hour. There aren't too many people who want to spend two hours working out. I think alternating days or doing some sort of a split-routine for strength training is the best way to go.

Q.) Is it better to exercise every part of the body on the same day or it better to focus on different muscle groups on different days?

A.) That depends on a person's goals and how many days per week they are willing to hit the gym. For someone who wants to body build, they are going to need a split routine and work certain body parts on certain days and, therefore, be at the gym more frequently. If I have someone who wants to spend the minimum number of days in the gym, then they are going to need to get it all in on those 2 or 3 days. The average person would see fantastic results working the entire body 3x per week (as well as controlling their diet). Again, that could be 3 days a week working all of the muscle groups, or 6 days a week doing a split-routine.

Q.) If someone doesn't have the time to spend hours cooking healthy meals, how can they still eat healthy?

A.) They can eat healthy by choosing the right foods (lean meat, fish or poultry, beans/legumes/nuts, whole grains, veggies and fruit and low or nonfat dairy). Choose to fill up on nonstarchy carbs (veggies and fruit) and add a serving or two of protein (men and women have different requirements). Pay attention to serving size. Everyone looks at the calories in a food, but do they pay attention to the serving size? If a person eats more than the serving size, they are getting more than what they read on the label. I teach my clients to get their non-starchy carbs, some whole grain starchy carbs, protein, Omega-3s, calcium, antioxidants and probiotics everyday. Other tips: Shop the perimeter of the grocery store (the processed stuff is usually in the middle of the store); Eat a rainbow everyday (foods of different colors offer a variety of nutrients); Eat breakfast like a king, lunch like a prince and dinner like a pauper (Too many people skip breakfast, eat lunch around noon or 1:00 then don't eat again until dinner then overeat because they are so hungry. This is a recipe for a metabolic disaster.) Unless the person has low blood sugar, they should just eat like a diabetic - or at least like someone trying to avoid getting diabetes.

Thank you Sherry...

If you would like to learn more about, Locke's Personal Fitness, their information will follow.

Locke's Personal Fitness, 88 Ft. Couch Road, Pittsburgh, PA 15241 (412) 835-5411 www.lockespersonalfitness.com Facebook Twitter

Sherry J. Locke
ACSM Certified Personal Trainer
Locke's Personal Fitness, Inc.
88 Ft. Couch Road
Pittsburgh, PA 15241
(412) 835-5411
www.lockespersonalfitness.com

Chapter (6)

PURE FIT CLUB

"Answers provided by Charles Defrancesco, Owner"

"Pure Fit Club is a different kind of fitness facility because we believe education should be the foundation of everyone's routine. Our partner Fit and Functional operates a <u>school for personal trainers</u> on site. This school provides Pure's staff with education and research which is free to all members.

Our trainers specialize in functional rehabilitation and using common, everyday movements to achieve exercise success. Whether it be weight-loss, muscle building, body toning, strength conditioning, or sports training, we are fully versed in every facet of exercise science. In fact, as director of education at NFPT, *our board of education headed the rewrite for the NFPT Accredited CPT credential. In addition, we have developed multiple specialty courses in cooperation with Fit and Functional, Next Level Speed and Westchester Sports & Wellness. All courses are nationally recognized and approved by some of the highest level organizations in the industry."* ~ Charles Defrancesco

Q.) What's a good way to find a reputable, trust-worthy personal trainer?

A.) This is very difficult because most people have no way to tell the difference between a good one and a bad one. You would think credentials would matter but in most cases the guys with the most degrees and certificates are not always best. Do not depend on the gym because even the biggest names you know hire based on sales and marketability and over look the education and experience. The best way would be through your doctor or look for trainers that have doctors you can call and reference. Most people take the cheapest guy because they think as long as they are certified or have a degree the trainer must be good. Call professional references not their regular clients, who of course will say good things. I attached an article I wrote on this.

Q.) Do people have to join the gym that their personal trainer belongs to, in order to hire them?

A.) In most cases a client has to join the gym to workout with a trainer who works there. The big gyms almost never let a non member train and if they do the session rate is ridiculously high. I have seen a few private gyms allow non members to train and studios almost never require membership fees. In some cases the gym just charges trainers a per session fee for clients they bring in. In my facilities I allow trainers to bring their own clients in without a membership and allow non membership training at the same rate as member sessions. For trainers outside clients we charge $25 for non members and $20 if they join, non members may only use the gym on scheduled session days.

Q.) Who should the average person talk to about which exercise program would be best for them?

A.) This is a great question to ask your doctor while reviewing your annual physical results. If you know a good trainer they can help you figure out all your needs and then set goals.

Q.) Are certain types of cardio workouts better than others?

A.) Yes. It all depends on your goal and what your limitations are. Usually interval training is the most beneficial but not everyone can do it. I find a mix of interval and low level cardio is easy to follow and can benefit everyone.

Q.) What's the difference between "aerobic" and "anaerobic" exercises?

A.) Aerobic is creating energy with oxygen during exercise. Anaerobic is creating energy without oxygen. Weight training and sprinting are anaerobic while walking or jogging is aerobic.

Q.) How long should people rest in between workouts?

A.) Recovery is the most important thing and nobody talks about it. You can only train as hard as you can recover. In a healthy individual, eating enough nutrients, stretching and getting 8 hours of sleep you can hit a muscle group every 72 hours and do a combination of interval and low level cardio 4-6 times per week depending on goals. As you get older you need more recovery workouts like stretching, foam rolling, yoga or low level cardio. Everyone needs at least 1 full day of rest and should never train when feeling sore or weak in that muscle group.

Q.) Should children lift weights?

 A.) Yes but under careful supervision and never super heavy. If they play sports they can exercise and stretch. I believe kids should focus on body weight exercises, basic movement mechanics and stretching before anything else. Light weights are usually good around age 8-10 but varies between individuals.

Q.) How accurate are the calorie counters on gym machines?

A.) If they do not take your lean body mass into account they are not very accurate at all. It's a good way to get an estimate.

Q. How important is nutrition if someone works out consistently?

A.) More important than anything because food is fuel and recovery.

Q.) Should a personal trainer know all of the medications someone is on? Why or why not?

A.) Yes because if there is ever a medical emergency the trainer needs that info and some meds effect heart rate and exercise intensity.

Q.) Should people with low blood sugar do anything differently before, during, or after a workout?

A.) Yes they need to figure out why it is low to begin with. In most cases the doctor will advise the patient to eat something before exercise to maintain proper levels during exercise. In addition the patient may be asked to carry hard candy or have access to juice if it drops too low.

Q.) Is it true that it's bad to eat too much fruit because of all of the sugar it contains?

A.) I hear this often and always get a laugh. I have never met someone who was fat or unhealthy from eating too much fruit. Some fruits do have high sugar levels but in my opinion it is natural and unprocessed. For diabetics there may be an issue but I don't see one for anyone else unless you are trying to compete as a body builder.

Q.) Is it true that exercise and a healthy diet can help reduce the chance of developing diabetes? If this is true, how can exercise and/or a good nutrition plan help prevent diabetes?

A.) Yes it is absolutely true and it also prevents a variety of other illnesses. People who eat well and exercise are usually not overweight and cleaner foods are less toxic. Building and maintaining muscle as we age will increase metabolism and basically stop the body from rusting like an old car. Healthy foods do not spike insulin and exercise will keep the body healthy and fit.

Society would rather believe there is nothing you can do and its all genetic so lets take drugs. Truth is in many cases poor diet and lack of exercise are the reason these things happen. Overweight people get sick and the stress of the bad food destroys the body's ability to function. I have seen many diabetics lose weight and change habits and all of a sudden they are doing well and either need less meds or none.

Q.) Most experts seem to all agree that nuts are very healthy, but they seem to have a lot of fat in them. Won't eating high fat foods like nuts make it more difficult to lose weight?

A.) They do have a lot of fat but it is good fat. Good fat actually removes bad fat and can be a great long term energy resource. Good fat builds muscle tissue and aids recovery. Beware because too much of anything isn't good and raw is better than roasted.

Thank you Charles...

If you would like to learn more about Pure Fitness Group, their information will follow.

Pure Fitness Group
1133 Westchester Ave Main Lobby
White Plains, NY 10604
also facilities in Rye and Greenwich
http://www.purefitclub.com/
Charles DeFrancesco 914 774 3644

Rymor Publishing Group

This page intentionally left blank

Chapter (7)

THE FITNESS CENTER AT THE MYERBERG

"Answers provided by Nicole Barr,
Director of Health & Fitness"

Nicole Barr has been in the Fitness Industry for over 7 years. Nicole began her Fitness career at Bally Total Fitness, as a Personal Trainer. Soon after, she started Fly-By Fitness, an In-Home Personal Training Company, based in the Baltimore, MD area. Along with her independent training company, Nicole is also Director of Health & Fitness at The Myerberg Fitness Center, located in Baltimore, MD. She is a Certified Personal Trainer (WITS), Certified Senior Fitness Specialist (NASM), and a Yoga Fit Instructor. Nicole specializes in weight loss/management and corrective exercise.

Q.) What are some questions that people should ask a personal trainer before hiring them?

A.) Most likely, any trainer working in a Fitness Center will have his/her Certification and have to maintain that Certification with additional continuing education credits every year or every couple of years. Most states do not require that Certified Trainers also have a degree in an exercise related field. The thing most clients don't realize is that a "Certification" can mean anything, these days. There are Certifications online for $50, where someone can answer 20 questions and be "Certified". My advice is to ask a Trainer where they got their Certification and then check either of these websites to make sure that Certification is listed as an accredited Certifying body: http://www.nbfe.org/about/affiliate/ or http://www.credentialingexcellence.org. That being said, Personal Training is not always about what education or training a person has, but his/her experience. I would suggest asking a Trainer how long he/she has been working as a Personal Trainer.

More experienced Trainers will have worked with more clients with a variety of goals, past injuries, and imbalances. More experience can mean that a Trainer might understand your wants and needs and how to attain them more clearly and precisely. Some Trainers just put a client through the motions, without any thought given to a client's body alignment and composition. That can be dangerous and detrimental to not only to your health and well-being, but it can hinder progress. For example, if your goal is to run a 5K, but your lower back causes you pain from time to time, an inexperienced trainer might immediately set you up on a running program and show you some stretches to help the back pain. That would be the "textbook" approach to reach your goal.

An experienced Personal Trainer would take the time to assess your body's posture, alignment, and watch how you walk to pinpoint why your back may be causing you problems. Knowing the source of the pain, a Trainer can create a corrective exercise program and then slowly introduce the 5K program, once the Trainer feels the client's body has adapted and is ready to begin. With that in mind, don't be discouraged if in the beginning, a Trainer might not have you doing 50 squats and pushups to get you "ripped". That could only lead to injury and keep you from reaching your goal all together.

Q.) What are some ways to verify the credentials/certifications of a personal trainer?

A.) In addition to the two websites I listed in my previous response, you can visit IDEAFit.com and search for Trainers in your area. The Trainers will list their credentials and IDEA Fit will verify them. So, you can be certain their Certifications are accurate and up-to-date.

Q.) Is it customary for a personal trainer to provide references of satisfied clients?

A.) Referrals are a Trainer's number one source of clients. A client's experience can really make or break a Trainer's career and therefore, most Trainers will include Testimonials on their website to advertise their clients' accomplishments. If you can't find any testimonials, don't be afraid to ask a Trainer to send some to you. Though the Trainer won't be able to provide contact info for any of his/her clients, the Trainer can compile some to share with you.

Q.) Are there ways to reduce recovery time or soreness between workouts, without taking supplements?

A.) In our Fitness Center, I witness so many members who come in, work out hard, and then leave immediately after without stretching. This is a MAJOR no-no! Soreness can set in even 20 minutes after a workout if stretching is not included at the end. Skipping stretching can lead to a long list of future injuries and pain, particularly in the knees, hips, and back. I want to begin by explaining the difference between a "stretch" and an "exercise". A stretch is static and done in a position that is held for at least 30 seconds. It is typically not performed repetitiously. For example, a right leg hamstring stretch would be performed lying on your back, using a stretching strap. The strap is placed behind the right foot and the leg is extended straight and the foot is lifted away from the floor, until you feel a slight pull in the back of the leg. The leg is held at that position for at least 30 seconds and the stretch is then repeated on the left leg. Slow, deep breathing is important when stretching to release any lingering tension in the muscle. If you're unsure of what kind of stretches would be best for your body, please speak with your Personal Trainer.

 Your Trainer might also introduce you to some Myo-Facial Release techniques to release muscle tension. With Myo-Facial Release, a foam roller or balls of various sizes are used to apply pressure to tender or sore muscles, until the muscle relaxes. It's very similar to techniques a masseuse might use, but it can be done on your own. Myo-Facial Release can help prevent soreness and help increase recovery time. You can also ask your Trainer about how to properly execute these techniques.

In addition to stretching and Myo-Facial Release, I recommend drinking plenty of fluids and having a small meal within an hour after working that includes high quality protein (fish, poultry, eggs, etc) and complex carbohydrate (banana, sweet potato) to replenish the body's nutrients and "feed" the muscles. During exercise, carbohydrates are depleted and the muscle fibers break down. During recovery, carbohydrates should be replaced and protein should be included to help repair and rebuild the muscle fibers, which results in stronger muscles. Sufficient recovery time is also very important. I recommend not working the same muscle group every day to give the muscles enough time to repair. A good idea is to have your Trainer create a program you can do on opposing days. For example, you could do exercises for the upper body on Monday and then exercises for the lower lody on Tuesday.

You should also rest your muscles longer when necessary. For example, if you performed Chest Presses on Monday and by Wednesday your chest is still sore to the touch, do some cardio (treadmill, bike, etc) and stretch the chest muscles. Avoid doing Chest Presses until the muscle is no longer sore to the touch.

Q.) Why don't crash diets work?

A.) I'm not a fan of the word "diet" at all! It's tied to negative connotations and a feeling "restriction". I find some of the most successful nutrition plans are the ones that are described as being "healing" for your body. If we think of nutrition as providing vitamins and nutrients to our bodies and not strictly for weight loss, we'll be more likely to stick with the healthier choices. Some studies tell us that taking a vitamin supplement will give us the daily vitamins we need while other studies say that the vitamin supplements do nothing, but act as a placebo. My theory is that if we get our vitamins from real food (the way nature had intended it), our bellies will break down the foods more efficiently and not only have access to the vitamins sooner, but the belly will spend less time fighting off foreign objects and can focus on repairing the body when it's needed the most.

 In a nutshell, getting vitamins from REAL food can boost our immune systems! As a rule of thumb, choose foods that are nutrient dense. A book I read recently that was really great at explaining how certain foods affect the body is "It Starts with Food" by Dallas & Melissa Hartwig. The book is based on a 30-Day belly healing plan, where certain foods are removed from the diet for 30 days, then slowly reintroduced. Approaching food in this way can help you learn how your body reacts to certain foods. After I followed the plan, I realized that beans and dairy had been upsetting my stomach all along. I also realized how much grains not only affected my weight, but my energy levels. I would've never known these things about my body if I had not cut them out entirely.

 I also learned how to get more of a variety of fruits and veggies in my diet and to cook more wholesome meals. For example, did you know that the amount of calcium in 1.5 cups of kale is equivalent to 1 cup of milk? Did you know that our bodies require Vitamin D (naturally found in fatty fish (salmon, sardines) and egg yolks) to absorb Calcium? Did you know our bodies need fat to absorb Calcium? Now, you can start to see just how important it is to get our vitamins the natural way - FOOD! My advice is to meet with a Registered Dietician to discuss your nutrition more in-depth and to stick with reputable sources for the latest research on nutrition. I like using the New England Journal of Medicine for any new research on diet and exercise.

Please be aware that most Trainers are not Nutritionists and more often than not will refer you to a Registered Dietician. Different states have different requirements for Registered Dieticians, so it's best to familiarize yourself with the qualifications.

Q.) If someone feels that their trainer is pushing them too hard, or not hard enough how should they handle this?

A.) As I mentioned previously, it is not uncommon for a Trainer to start with corrective exercises in the beginning to fix imbalances, weaknesses, and postural alignment issues. Your Trainer should explain why he/she is having you do certain exercises, so you can understand.

When I first started Training, I thought it was my job to push my clients to the max! As the years went on, I learned that is definitely NOT the way to train my clients nor myself. I now design programs, based on a few factors: Is this exercise appropriate for my client? Will this exercise assist or hinder my client's posture? Will this exercise help or aggravate any previous injuries or medical conditions?

It is important to get the heart rate within it's appropriate training zones for sufficient cardio exercise, which may mean working harder or less hard, depending on your heart rate, which a Trainer can help you figure out. As for strength training, it is a good idea to push yourself, but not to the point where you're performing the exercise incorrectly or losing form. For example, when doing squats, pay attention to your back and knees. If at any moment your lower back starts to round or knees start to buckle in, you've probably reach your max and should move on to the next exercise. If at any point, you feel pain, be sure to ask your Trainer to check your form or ask for a modified exercise. Also, don't be afraid to be open with your trainer and tell him/her how you're feeling at any moment. I ask my clients quite frequently "Are you Ok?" and "How are you doing?"

Q.) How does someone tone up and lose fat under their arms and around their triceps?

A.) Losing fat always starts with good nutrition (75% of the battle!) and a well crafted cardio and strength training program that includes all major muscle groups. Unless you're already lean to begin with, spot training to lose weight in a specific area does not work. Our bodies are genetically predisposed to lose and gain in certain areas faster than others. Therefore, attention has to be given to all parts of the body to see results. We can always include tricep exercises in our workouts, but don't skimp on all the other areas, like the legs, chest, back, and core. Stick to dynamic exercises (ex squats with back row, lunges w/ chest press) that use multiple muscle groups to maximize energy output. Also, try minimizing rest between exercises. You'll burn more calories the way!

Another thing to know about burning fat is that doing interval cardio workouts will always burn more calories than working out at a steady speed/resistance. There are numerous studies that prove that to be true! For example, using the "Interval" program on the elliptical will burn more calories than staying steady at a 3.0 resistance level.

Q.) For people who are always tired, won't working out make them feel like they have even less energy?

A.) If your nutrition is good and balanced, the exercise should actually increase energy. The hardest part is always getting started, but once you get on the treadmill and start moving, the body will start to release endorphins and you'll not only get an increase in general mood, but you'll feel more awake and rejuvenated! It may make you sleepier just before bed, but that's what most of us want! We want a good night's sleep and exercise can help.

Q.) What's the difference between "good carbs" and "bad carbs"?

A.) Though this is a question best answered by a Registered Dietician, it's no mystery to us what is "good" and "bad" carbs. For a refresher, "good" carbs are typically found in natural foods with minimal processing, like fruits and veggies. A good rule of thumb is that "good" carbs come from the produce section. "Bad carbs" are typically processed, multi-ingredient foods that can be found in the "snacks" and "packaged goods" aisles. Things like cookies, bread, cakes, muffins, and even cereal can be considered "bad" carbs. I tell most of my clients that there are no vitamins and nutrients in granola or cereals that can't be found in fruits, veggies, and lean meats. In fact, I refer to grains (pasta, rice, bread, oatmeal, etc) as empty calories. Those items are high in calories, but really don't payoff in the amount of nutrients and vitamins they provide. Why not go with a cup of mixed fruit (pineapple, strawberries, and blueberries) and get less calories and more vitamins and nutrients than a bowl of cereal?! Sounds like a good deal to me!

Q.) Is it true that stress makes people gain weight? What is the truth, if any, behind this?

A.) I have several clients who suffer from stress and it shows. Typically, people who have trouble keeping their stress under control carry excess weight in the belly area. This is due to increased levels of cortisol. Cortisol is known as "the stress hormone" because it's secreted in higher levels during the body's "fight or flight" response to stress. Higher and more prolonged levels of cortisol in the bloodstream causes, not only things like suppressed thyroid function and higher blood pressure, but also causes increased abdominal fat. Carrying excess abdominal fat has also been linked to increase in risk for heart attacks and stroke.

The best way to overcome stress is to eat a balanced diet that includes plenty of fruits, veggies, and lean means and exercising daily. Even 30 minutes on the treadmill can boost your mood immensely. You could also try a Yoga or Tai Chi class, which both practice breathing, stretching, and strengthening. The classes will teach the body how to manage high-stress situations by training the mind to release and relax. A relaxed mind leads to a relaxed body and freedom from ourselves.

Other techniques I've used to manage stress include listening to music that makes me feel happy, writing in a journal, and just doing some deep breathing, allowing my belly to fill up with air. One of the best ways to relieve stress? Sex! Enjoy.

Q.) Fish seems to have a lot of fat in it. Will people gain weight if they eat too much fish?

A.) Blasphemy! Fish is one of the best sources of Vitamin D and one of the few ways to get it naturally. Also, it's important to know that fat is not the enemy. Studies show that managing weight really comes down to calories and not fat. Fat is actually a very important part of our diet. It helps our bodies digest and absorb Vitamins A, D, E, and K. Fat also helps us maintain healthy skin and hair, maintains our body temperature, and promotes healthy cell function. One of fat's most important roles is to provide energy for our bodies. So, enjoy the fat and watch the calories.

Q.) If someone is a heavy smoker, should their workout routine be adjusted at all? If so, how?

A.) As long as a person is cleared by their doctor to exercise, I would suggest a normal exercise routine, such as walking on the treadmill or using the bike or stepper and increasing time and intensity when their body is ready. I would also suggest researching ways to break the habit of smoking, as continuing to smoke while starting an exercise program is counterproductive.

Q.) Is there any truth to the claim that exercise can help improve brain function and/or mental focus? If yes, how?

A.) Absolutely! In a recent study, it was concluded that people in their seventies who participated in more physical exercise had less brain shrinkage and other signs of aging in the brain than those who were less physically active. Exercise is used to help treat patients with Alzheimer's, as well. This is most likely due to the fact that exercise increases blood flow throughout the body and the brain. I personally find that I am my most creative self when I am working out. I come up with some great ideas on the elliptical!

Q.) What are the biggest mistakes people make when hiring a personal trainer?

A.) I think more often than not, new Personal Training clients think of a Trainer as a "magic pill". Though Trainers are experienced and very knowledgeable in how to achieve client's goals, it's important for clients to know that it starts with them. A client has to be not only willing to learn, but also committed to themselves. I know some Trainers who will turn clients away if they feel they're not ready mentally or continually fail to follow a plan and stay on track. So, just be sure you're mentally prepared to make the commitment before working with a Trainer. That way, you're sure to see results and not just throwing money into wind!

Q.) What can people do to avoid back injuries when they're lifting weights?

A.) It's all about posture and form! It's a good idea to consult a Trainer to make sure your form is correct.

There are a few things to keep in mind when performing an upper body exercise:

1. Typically, you'll want to stand with feet hip distance apart.

2. Keep chest open and shoulders down and back (retracted).

3. Keep naval pulled in to spine, so the abdominals stay contracted.

4. Exhale as you lift, press, or pull (*general rule of thumb: exhale during the hard parts).

5. If your goal is to lose weight and you lose proper form after a few repetitions, consider decreasing the weight. You should be able to do 12-15 repetitions with good form.

Thank you Nicole...

If you would like to learn more about The Fitness Center at The Myerberg, their information will follow.

Nicole Barr
Certified Personal Trainer & Corrective Exercise Specialist

Business #1:
Fitness Center at The Myerberg | Director of Health & Fitness
3101 Fallstaff Rd., Baltimore, MD 21209
Phone: 410-358-6856
Email: myerbergfitnesscenter@gmail.com
Website: http://www.myerbergseniorcenter.org

Business #2:
Fly-By Fitness (Owner)| Home Personal Training
Phone: 410-205-9360
Email: info@fly-byfitness.com
Website: www.fly-byfitness.com
Blog: http://theroot.fly-byfitness.com/

Rymor Publishing Group

This page intentionally left blank

Chapter (8)

TAYLOR CARPENTER PERSONAL TRAINING, LLC

"Answers provided by Taylor Carpenter, Founder"

Taylor Carpenter Personal Training LLC is located at a 1250 sq ft state of the art studio located in the Ballantyne area of Charlotte, NC. I've been certified as a personal trainer & corrective exercise specialist by the National Academy of Sports Medicine.

"I really enjoy working one on one with clients and I'm the only facility in the area that offers truly private personal training where at certain times a client can have my facility all to themselves while working with their trainer. Group training & Saturday Fitness classes are also currently two other options for potential clients in addition to the premier one on one training service. I encourage all my clients to utilize the free calorie counting website & app "My Fitness Pal" to effectively let me offer them nutritional guidance. Major brand name supplements are also available to my clients with a well below retail discount (BSN, Cytosport, Dymatize, Controlled Labs, Optimum Nutrition, etc). In the near future I hope to offer a variety of specialty classes teaching people newer techniques such as self myofascial release, suspension training, etc..." ~Taylor Carpenter

Q.) How much will it cost to hire a personal trainer?

A.) The cost of a personal trainer should vary highly based on where you live and the cost of living just as anything else. I'd guess the average rate for an experienced trainer would be between $50-$70.00. Where your trainer works is also a consideration that would reflect upon the price. Many trainers just starting out may provide in home training, apartment training, etc which I've seen many advertise for about $25 a session. If you're looking for a trainer in a box gym or a trainer who has their own studio expect to pay closer to the $70-$80 per hour range. The experience level is higher and the trainer's overhead is higher so the client will typically have a higher cost. Experience should never be overlooked though, many certifications are relatively easy to obtain and just because your trainer has an impressive physique does not necessarily mean they know the proper mechanics, or even more so, what's ideal for you and your situation.

My rates are based on how many times per week a person works out with me. The more sessions per week, the lower the session rate. Usually if the client makes a larger commitment then the trainer will provide a better deal. I'd recommend clients be cautious before entering an extremely long term rate and read your contract very carefully!

Q.) How long should a personal training session last?

A.) It really depends on the client, their goals, and their current fitness level. 30 minute sessions are becoming more and more prevalent around the country because they're almost half the price of a full hour session. I've worked with clients who really have a hard time with 30 minutes when they get started and then others who felt 45 minutes was the perfect time frame from the jump.

I teach clients early on how they should warm up and cool down, which could essentially be about 20 minutes of your work out. They come early to perform that while I'm finishing up with my previous client. I'm not having them pay to do something they're really capable of doing on their own.

How much instruction a client needs, whether the client is battling or recovering from injury, what type of phase they're on in their training program are all factors that would determine what's appropriate for the client. Everyone has different needs.

Q.) Is it better to workout for a long period of time at a low intensity or a short period of time at a high intensity?

A.) This is also dependent upon an individual's needs. I would advise everyone to workout at an intensity they are capable of sticking with. Not everyone loves working out if their first encounter with training is so rapid that their sweating profusely, having a hard time catching their breath and getting beat down to exhaustion they're probably not going to stick with it too long.

On the other hand you have the gym rat who refuses to train any other way. It needs to be enjoyable (as much as it can be) so it becomes a regular part of your life. As a trainer, you try to find that intensity and slowly push the clients a little beyond without burning them out.

Q.) How do people get rid of loose skin after weight loss?

A.) As you improve your diet and exercising consistency your body composition will positively change. As you add on more lean muscle mass and burn off fat your body will positively change. However, in many cases with significant weight loss, the skin has been excessively stretched and the only thing that can be done to fix the hanging excess skin is surgery.

Q.) How do people measure their heart rate?

A.) The National Academy of Sports Medicine teaches us to take your resting heart rate in the morning immediately upon waking. Many factors can affect your heart rate so its best to take measurement 3-4 days in a row and average the results.

There are many heart rate monitors available at your local sports authority or dicks sporting goods if you'd like a reading during your workout or post workout. Usually the more expensive means the more effective.

I've never used an app on my phone for testing heart rate but I would assume by now there would have to be one on iPhone and Android for measuring your heart rate as well.

Q.) Why is it that, no matter how much cardio some people do, they still can't lose weight?

A.) In some cases it could be a medical issue. In majority of cases it's because the individual is consuming more calories then they are burning. Calories in vs Calories out. In order to lose weight you have to be using more calories than you're eating. I use myfitnesspal.com to log my food, its free & an excellent resource that you can use online or on your phone. When you see the macronutrients (protein, carbs, fat) and calorie value of what you're eating I really think it helps you learn a lot.

Q.) Do men lose weight faster than women?

A.) Some do, some don't. Everyone has a different metabolic rate, different diet, different workout routine, different schedule, different levels of stress, different amounts of sleep, etc...If everything was equal and a case study was done on this question I would think it would be a toss up based on the individuals that just so happened to be chosen. Everyone will follow a different path to reach their goal.

Q.) Is there an ideal time of day to workout?

A.) Yes, a time when you will get it done! Whether you workout in the mornings or in the evening it really doesn't matter...it's a personal preference. I do think it would be ideal to find a set and consistent time if your schedule allows. I see the most success when people schedule their workouts, make no excuses and do the same with their meal planning. Book them like you would a meeting at work and don't let anything interfere.
If you'd rather hit the snooze button then get up for your workout, trying training at lunch or after work. If you're job makes

you too tired after a long hard day's work...try the AM. Just find the best time that works for you.

Q.) Is aerobic walking as healthy as jogging or running?

A.) It can be...Walking, hiking, jogging, sprinting, rowing, weightlifting, cross training, recreational sports, etc...They're all great. Any movement is great for you!

However, different things are better for different people. People significantly overweight probably shouldn't be sprinting around slamming 300lbs onto their joints. Anyone with joint issues should avoid very high impact exercise & movements as it could do more harm than good. You've got to look at the individual to decide what's best for them at that particular point in their life but movement in general is much healthier than sitting still.

Q.) Can people use an exercise ball if they are overweight or obese?

A.) Most people can use a Swiss ball/exercise ball.....However, being that it's an unstable tool it should always be viewed at as a progression and not a starting point. Progressions should always begin in a stable environment before proceeding to an unstable one.

Q.) Is it bad to eat right before going to bed? Why or why not?

A.) No. As mentioned above, weight loss or weight gain comes from calories in vs calories out. Choose your goal and consume your caloric intake accordingly. Telling people not to eat before bed I believe was started to prevent people from overeating and binging at night. Everyone who has fitness goals needs to log their food and view that as their daily budget. Stay within your budget.
Q.) What are some tips that people should keep in mind, for practicing good form during their workouts?

A.) Google "hip hinge" or visit the ACE website at http://www.acefitness.org/acefit/fitness_programs_exercise_library_details.aspx?exerciseid=33

This a neat little exercise I found a while back that really helps protect your back. All you will need is a broom stick handle, a long ruler, or some very light weight pole. Common compensations trainers see are rounded shoulders, protruding head, arching of the low back, rounding of the low back. The hip hinge with a broom stick is an excellent test to see where you're at and what area of the body may be out of line.

Another observation you can make in the gym by yourself is to pay attention to your leg movement during squats, lunges, step ups, jumping, etc...Make sure the knee remains in line with your foot. If your leg is wobbling from side to side then you may be using too much weight or compensations are present that need to be addressed.

Q.) Can someone still lose weight if they split their workouts throughout the day?

A.) Calories in vs calories out again. It's a definite possibility, if that's what an individual's schedule requires that's how it has to be done. I'd prefer to train once a day, I'd prefer my clients train once a day but that's not possible for everyone. With work, kids, and a variety of obligations people have nowadays it may be necessary to split workouts. I don't think it's the ideal situation but goals can most definitely be reached.

Thank you Taylor...

If you would like to learn more about, Taylor Carpenter Personal Training, LLC, their information will follow.

Taylor Carpenter
17232 Lancaster Hwy, Suite 111
Charlotte NC, 28277

(704) 618-5853
taylorcarpenter@gmail.com
http://www.taylorcarpenter-pt.com
https://www.facebook.com/charlottetrainer

National Academy of Sports Medicine
Certified Personal Trainer & Corrective Exercise Specialist
(C) 704-618-5853
http://www.taylorcarpenter-pt.com
https://www.facebook.com/charlottetrainer

Rymor Publishing Group

This page intentionally left blank

Chapter (9)

SALDARE BODY THERAPHY & WELLNESS STUDIO

"Answers provided by Jennifer Menzer, Owner"

"Saldare Body Therapy offers a modern yet traditional approach in assisting our clients in improving their overall quality of life by incorporating individualized health, wellness, exercise and nutrition into your everyday lifestyle. Our services include personal and small group fitness training, holistic nutrition and health coaching, pilates and yoga instruction and an in-house physical rehabilitation therapist. In addition to our health and wellness services we also offer a menu of relaxing spa services including esthetics and skincare, therapeutic massage and acupuncture. Come visit us and discover the rewards of taking the time to nourish the body, mind, and spirit." ~Jennifer Menzer

Q.) Is there a difference between "cardio" and "aerobic"? If there is, what's the difference?

A.) The difference between cardio and aerobic is mostly semantics. Aerobic exercises promote a greater oxygen intake while cardiovascular exercises promote a greater heart rate. One always accompanies the other, but they are in fact two separate things.

Q.) Can sit-ups help people lose belly fat? Why do some people do thousands of sit-ups and they still don't lose any belly fat?

A.) Abs are 100% nutrition. I hate to be the one to burst the bubble, but no matter how hard we strengthen and tone our abdominal muscles, if we have a layer of fat covering them, then they will not be visible. To shed belly fat we need to have a clean diet of fruits, vegetables, lean protein, whole grains and avoid refined carbohydrates, sugar, alcohol and saturated fats.

Q.) What are some factors that impact people's metabolism?

A.) Metabolism is impacted by both exercise *and* diet. Cardiovascular exercise and resistance training will work to decrease fat and increase lean muscle mass which burns calories at a higher rate than fat. A diet rich in protein, fiber, essential fatty acids, vitamins and minerals will boost metabolism and your body will use the calories much more efficiently.

Q.) What can people do to stay motivated, after they've started a workout program?

A.) I would recommend everyone meet with a personal trainer for at least three sessions. This will provide a program that is individualized to their specific goals, will increase the effectiveness of the exercises due to ensuring proper form, and will decrease potential for injury. You also work harder with a trainer. Let's face it; we work harder when someone is cheering us on and encouraging us to do "just one more rep". Other things that help to stay motivated include a great mix on the iPod, working out with a friend, group classes and keeping a calendar up that tracks the number of times you've gone to the gym in the month.

Q.) If someone enjoys drinking alcohol in moderation, how often can they indulge without feeling guilty or undoing all the progress they made with their trainer?

A.) I encourage my clients to take on a 90/10 approach. 90% of the time they engage in clean eating which unfortunately does not include alcohol. The other 10% they are encouraged to eat and drink what they enjoy without worrying about the nutrient density. Based on that, I usually recommend a range of one to three glasses of red wine or vodka and sodas a week. If you want to trade those in for margaritas or fancy martinis, then you'll need to make up for it the following week! :)

Q.) If someone has a personal trainer, do they also need a nutritionist?

A.) As a personal trainer and a health and nutrition coach I recommend someone have the opportunity to have as many resources as possible to achieve the happiest most vibrant life and meet their goals.

Q.) What are the differences between a personal trainer and a nutritionist?

A.) The difference between the two are in the professional certifications. A nutritionist or a health coach seeks to educate the client and support them as they improve the nutrient density of foods they choose to consume, and achieve or maintain a healthy body weight. In addition, health coaches also promote and support healthy lifestyle choices such as exercise, decreased stress, and an enjoyable social and family life. They would not however, design a cardiovascular or strength training program for the client. A personal trainer assesses the clients overall cardiovascular endurance, strength, flexibility, and limitations and designs an individualized fitness program that supports the client's goals. Trainers encourage clients to adapt to a clean living diet and can make general recommendations, but cannot design an individualized meal plan or promote supplements.

Q.) What should people look out for when joining a gym?

A.) I cannot say that there are definitive things to look out for there are things I would recommend. Seek out a few gyms in the area and see which one feels the most comfortable and offers the amenities that are a definite on your list. Most importantly, make sure it is either close to work or home so you have no excuses getting there!

Q.) When it comes to working out, there seems to be a lot of conflicting information out there. How can people know what advice is good and what is not?

A.) Because everybody's body is different what may work wonders for one person may not be good for someone and in fact produce negative results. This is where I would recommend doing your own research. Good sources of information can be found online. I refer to the ACSM (American College of Sports Medicine) guidelines and sites from some of the experts in the field.

Q.) How should someone's age be taken into consideration, when starting a new exercise program?

A.) Age is important when starting a new exercise program, but it is only one part of the whole equation. We also need to take fitness level, injuries/limitations and body fat into account at the time of designing the program. I have an advanced 63 year old client that can maintain the suggested heart rate of a 25 year old and a de-conditioned client who is in her 20's, has excess body fat and cannot yet reach the base level of her suggested aerobic heart rate zone.

Q.) Does weight training cause people to lose flexibility?

A.) Yes and no. Yes because we are shortening the muscles and making microscopic tears to them in hopes that they will rest, repair and rebuild stronger. No because we do develop flexibility specific to the exercises we perform over time with weight training. Ideally, we should foam roll before a strength workout, and stretch after a strength workout to maintain our flexibility. Throw some yoga, massage, or facilitated stretching in there and the outcome will be even greater!

Q.) If someone can only workout once a week, should they even bother?

A.) Yes! One day is better than none, plus it helps to build a healthy habit that may then turn into two days based on the physical and emotional rewards exercise provides.

Q.) If someone also does yoga, should they workout on the same day that they have their yoga class?

A.) This depends on the person and their fitness level and goals. I personally don't see a problem doing something else before or after yoga as long as the person remembers to stay present and focused and to listen to their body.

Thank you Jennifer...

If you would like to learn more about, Saldare Body Therapy & Wellness Studio, their information will follow.

Jennifer Menzer
Saldare Body Therapy & Wellness Studio
 12 Clarendon St Boston, MA 02116
 www.saldarespa.com or www.bostonhealthcoaches.com
(617) 423-2722
 jenn@saldarespa.com
 Like us on Facebook too.

This page intentionally left blank

Chapter (10)

SIMPLE FITNESS

"Answers provided by Elina Davis, Owner"

"I'm a certified personal trainer & pilates instructor who loves helping people. I either travel to people's homes or they travel to me. Also, in January I've started teaching beginner's and intermediate mat pilates classes at Manchester. I do have an extensive fitness background and offers all kinds of cardiovascular and resistance training, such as: circuit style workouts, interval training and plyometrics. When it comes to resistance training, I utilize free weights, resistance bands, stability and medicine balls.

However, if you ask me what are the 2 things you are best at; it would be help with a lifestyle change and working with people with past or current injuries. I used to be 30 pounds heavier 9 years ago and I've developed my own system for people who would love to stay in shape and be healthy and still enjoy their food. The system is very flexible and can be easily customized for anybody. Also, it is sustainable and doesn't require hours per day in a gym or huge investment in groceries.

Due to the fact that I have been active majority of my life, I had to learn how to work out to prevent injuries and actually make your body healthier instead of exhausting it. I love helping people so I constantly educate myself on topic of injury rehabilitation and look for exercises and stretches which can be done by people with current or past injuries. I have experience working with people with arthritis, back problems and people who had knee reconstruction surgery done." ~Elina Davis

Q.) What should someone look for in a good health club/gym?

A.) A good health club/gym is the one which matches your goals, personality, work schedule, fitness level and workout habits as close as possible. I know a lot of people who have a lot of troubles with finding a gym which really works for them. And I think there are 2 reasons for it: 1) Is that some people don't exactly know what they are looking for when it comes to picking a gym; 2) They expect (want) too much from a gym.

Before picking a gym, I advise you to ask yourself the following questions:

1) If a gym is close enough to my house/ place of work?

2) If they have everything I need to successfully perform my workouts there? So, if you generally do a lot of cardiovascular activity, check the gym's cardio zone to make sure it matches your needs.

3) Do they have friendly and professional staff?

4) Do they take good care of the gym? Basically, you need to pay attention to how clean a gym is and if they have good ventilation, so, you won't be dying from overheating while running on a treadmill.

5) Do they have extra space where you can work out alone and if this space is generally not crowded? I'm talking about women's rooms or rooms for group classes.
6) If the equipment in the gym is in a good condition.

7) If there is enough space in the gym.

8) If they make you sign a year agreement, and if you are ok with that.

9) If they have a personal trainer or nutritionist on staff.

It is important, if you are a beginner and need somebody to guide you. Finally, if the gym offers good group classes, which you might be interested in. As you can see, it is a big list and probably some things won't apply to you, but I've tried to make it as comprehensive as possible.

And always remember, if you are not able to find the gym which works for you, you can always workout at home. It does require some planning, and you probably will have to invest in some good workout dvd's, in – home personal trainer and/or some equipment but it is a feasible option.

Q.) Is there an "ideal" time of day to workout?

A.) You know, when it comes to nutrition or fitness, it seems as if there is always a polar opposite view on a particular topic. For example, about a year ago, I decided to do some research on the squat. More specifically, I wanted to know if people with arthritis should do squats or avoid them. Long story short, some sources said that squats are an absolute no – no for people with arthritis and the other one said that it is a very beneficial exercise.

So, I've learned to use my own judgment and most importantly, treat myself and every client as an individual. We are all different. It applies to the way our body works and to the way our daily lives are set up.

If you are struggling with making a decision on when to work out, I advise you to consider the following things:

 1) your energy levels during the day. Some people feel more energetic in the mornings and others are more productive during the afternoon or evening hours. So, try to work out when you have a lot of energy, so you can perform better and last longer.

 2) Your typical work schedule during the day. If you work a lot of hours and your schedule is hectic, always have a simple and short

workout plan on you and work out wherever you have an opportunity, even if you just do it for 10 minutes at a time, it still much better than nothing.

3) Your nutrition during a particular day. Let's say, it is Saturday and you are going to have a dessert at dinner, it would be good if you schedule your workout 1 – 2 hours before the dinner or shortly after it, so it will help you to minimize the damage which cake causes to your health and looks.

So, I don't believe that there is such thing as ideal time for working out, but there is such thing as whatever works for as a particular individual.

Q.) If someone spent the day doing something very strenuous like mountain biking or hiking for an entire day, should they take a day off before working out or does the other activity not count as a real workout?

A.) It is a bit tricky question, because there are a lot of factors which need to be taken into consideration. Things like fitness level, workout load during a typical week, general lifestyle, stress levels and specific fitness goals will affect the answer. So, for example, if a person generally works at the desk, doesn't move a lot or even exercise regularly and his or her goal is start being active on a regular basis, a strenuous activity like hiking for an entire day should be considered as a real workout and a person should take a day off after doing it. I really think that a day off is a necessity in this case just because you don't want somebody to burn out or be too sore next day because if they are sore or burnt out, they might as well just quit working out all together.

However, if a person is very athletic, didn't workout too much this particular week, he or she might workout the next day. But just in case, I would still try to do something completely different to prevent overuse syndrome in a long term. So, if a person did hiking, I would do some resistance training for upper body the next day to give my lower body a break.

Q.) Is it true that genetics or body physiology make it impossible for some people to get in shape?

A.) No, this is definitely false. However, in some cases it may be harder for certain people to achieve certain fitness goals. But harder doesn't mean impossible. For example, I'm rather a big boned girl and it is easier for me to gain muscle mass than to lose weight. I also have most of my fat stored in my legs and my mother, grandmother and grand – grandmother has absolutely the same body type as mine. Does it mean that I will never be able to have skinny legs and a small tush because of my genetics? No, but it does mean that I have to work extremely hard for it to happen. So, honestly, at that point I'm not going to try to have the skinniest legs on the planet, but I will still have them in decent shape. They will, probably will, never be the best part of my body, but I will do my best to keep them in shape and will focus on appreciating other areas of my body, like my flat stomach for example.

It is all about keeping a balance between our desire to change our nature and obsessing too much about it.

Q.) How can people accurately determine how many calories they burn during a workout?

A.) I'm going to say something controversial, but I don't believe that there is a reliable way to measure the calories you burn during the workout. Of course, there are different devices which you can use to do it, but they still have some margin of error. Also, I do think that there are a lot of factors which affect your calories expenditure during the workout and none of the tools can take all of them into consideration. Let's say even if the device will take into consideration how much you ate today, it won't necessarily know what exactly you ate and all foods are not created equal from a nutrition standpoint and thus will affect differently your calories expenditure during the workout.

However, I'm personally not a fan of counting calories when it comes to working out. I don't think it is the most reliable criteria to use if you try to measure the effectiveness of your workout.

The more important thing is intensity. I know a lot of people, including myself who can have a short but intense training session (let's say do running interval for 20 minutes), don't burn so many calories during it, but see better results than somebody who walked for couple of hours and burned a lot. I think it has to do with the fact that when your workout intensely, you shock your body and thus it changes it and over time helps you speed up the metabolism even after workout is done sometimes.
Also, let be honest here. Sometimes when you think that you've burnt a lot of calories, you let yourself slip with your diet and thus sabotage yourself.

Thus, I think that counting calories when it comes to diet (or simply watching your portion sizes) is much more important that counting calories when working out especially considering the fact that it is very hard to precisely measure it.

Q.) What is the "fat burning zone" that trainers often refer to?

A.) Fat burning zone is a term closely connected with your target heart rate. It can be a bit confusing and I will try my best to explain it. Before you start a new workout routine and/or a diet, you need to know exactly what you are trying to achieve. Your goal should be really specific and measurable. So, let say you've decided to decrease your body fat percentage by 5 percent in the next 3 months or so. Then, you should come up with a good nutrition, cardiovascular plan and resistance training plan which will match this goal. Then, you should learn what your maximum heart rate is. It is very easy. If you are man, you subtract your age from 220 and if you are a woman, then you subtract your age from 226. Then, when you do your cardio, you make sure that you stay within the range for fat burning zone which is 60 to 70 percent of maximum heart rate. If you stay within this range and your goal is to decrease your body fat percentage, combined with a diet and good resistance training plan, you will definitely be able to achieve your goals. Fat burning zone is named this way because majority of calories burned in it comes from fat (about 85%) in comparison with Endurance training zone in which only 15% of calories burned come from fat.

So, as you can see your goal is to match your fitness goal with an appropriate training zone to help you achieve the best possible results.

Q.) How can people tell if they're doing enough exercise or exercising intensely enough?

A.) As a personal trainer, I get asked this question a lot. Based on my experience, the answer is very simple: if you are able to achieve your fitness goals with a particular workout plan then you are doing enough exercise, and exercising intensely enough.

For example, you really would like to take off a couple of inches of your waistline so you will feel more confident in a swimsuit. So, you decide to run 3 – 4 times per week around the neighborhood for 20 – 30 minutes at time (presuming that diet stays the same) but inches are still not going anywhere. It means that you are not doing enough exercise or exercising intensely enough to achieve this particular goal.
Of course, there are other factors which needs to be taken into consideration like diet for example, but based on experience, if a person are doing enough exercise or exercise intensely enough, he/she will still be able to at least partially achieve a specific fitness goal even if he/she doesn't change the diet.

Q.) How can personal trainers design programs for people with arthritis, who are unable to perform certain common exercises?

A.) I really think this question was made for me, because I do work with people who either have or had arthritis or have serious knee and back problems. Currently, I have a long – term senior client who has arthritis in both of his knees. So, before I've started making a workout routine for him, I made sure to ask him:

1) What kind of arthritis and how severe it is?

2) How long has he had it.

3) If there are any specific activities and/or exercises which aggravate it or make it feel better?

4) If he takes medication for it?

5) What his doctor thinks about his arthritis and working out?

6) If he tried physical therapy and what worked for him?

Then, I did some research and found out that when it comes to making a program for people with arthritis the following things need to be considered and included into the workout:

1) Strength moves for hamstrings, hip adductors, abductors, glutes and quads. I've used a combination of pilates, moves and squats to achieve this goal.

2) All the moves have to be done slow and under control to ensure proper form. When it comes to moves like squats, it should be a partial squat with either no weight or light weight and regular squats can be replaced with a chair pose from yoga, when you squat a little bit and just hold the position for a little bit instead of going up and down.

3) Low – impact cardio should be included to warm – up the body and to help the body bring oxygen and blood to the muscles.

4) At least a third of the workout should be devoted to stretching and flexibility training. Hamstring muscles, hip flexor muscles and quadriceps must be stretched every workout and stretches from yoga, physical therapy and assisted stretches can be very helpful but have to be done carefully to ensure safety.

5) Finally, when it comes to people with arthritis or back problems, I try to make them stand up and go down on the floor as less as possible. So, generally, we do all standing up exercises first, and then we go on the floor to do some mat exercises, and still stay on the floor for assisted stretching.

Q.) How can people prevent joint injuries or sore joints when lifting weights?

A.) In general, any physical activity processes some risk so even if you do everything right, it doesn't guarantee that you won't get injured, because every single body is different and nobody exactly knows how each individual's body will respond to exercise, but here are a couple of things which can help you to minimize the risk of injuring your joints and manage your soreness when lifting weights:

1. Always warm – up before starting your work out. You can do some light cardiovascular activity like walking on a treadmill, or you can do some warm – up sets (more reps, no weights or light weights).

2. Always cool down after a workout by stretching all the major muscle groups you worked on during your weight – lifting session. If you prefer to do cardio after your weight – training session, stretch after you are done with you cardio workout.

3. Always do each exercise with a proper form. I would say even more, try to do every single rep of every single exercise with a proper form because it doesn't always take many reps to injury yourself especially if you lift heavy.

4. Never do exercises which you don't know how to do properly. There are a lot of exercises, which requires many attempts to master them or need to be shown by somebody. So, if you are not sure, don't do it.

5. Never take more weight than your body can handle. If you can't perform an exercise with a proper form, lower the weight.

6. Make sure that you give your muscles enough time to recover. Even if you can't sleep at nights without thinking about a toned butt, for example, it doesn't mean that you have to train it every day and increase your chances for injury.

7. Don't over train. Be patient, consistent and train hard and results will come.

8. Make sure to take vitamins and take enough protein and carbohydrates to help your body restore after your weight – training sessions.

Thank you Elina...

If you would like to learn more about, Simple Fitness, their information will follow.

Elina Davis (Certified personal trainer & Pilates Instructor):

Cell: 603. 219. 4826
Email: elinadavis86@gmail.com
Facebook: https://www.facebook.com/ElinaTheTrainer
Website: nhpersonaltrainer.com
For pilates classes schedule and location:
Livingroomwellness.com
https://www.facebook.com/LivingRoomWellnessCenter?fref=ts
or contact me via cell or email for more info or to schedule a private pilates or personal training session.

Chapter (11)

OFFICIAL FITNESS PRO

*"Answers provided by Jeremy L Dancy,
Owner & Chief Executive Officer"*

Official FitnessPro also known as OFP was founded in 2006. At OFP we approach fitness in a different manner from our competition. Our experts focus their attention in specific areas of exercise. We have a team approach, consulting with each other regularly to perpetuate results, and provide the best customer service possible. We offer two types of personal training programs based on hands on accountability for aggressive goals or professional guidance for fitness veterans and beginners looking to develop a program specific to their needs. We have three locations on the west side of Cleveland. We offer specialized personal training programs in the areas of youth fitness, strength & conditioning, therapeutic exercise, and weight management.

Q.) Is it a good idea to workout when feeling mentally stressed? Why or why not?

A.) Yes it is a good idea for people to workout while feeling mentally stressed. Exercise give people a chance to get more involved with themselves and escape the trials and tribulations of the real world. Not to mention that the physical demands on the body from exercise stimulates endorphins and raises serotonin levels within the body. Serotonin is the main hormone responsible for enhancing calm and lowering stress.

Q.) Is it safe for obese people to lift weights?

A.) People who are obese need to be properly screened before beginning an exercise program. It can be safe or unsafe depending on the individual's limitations. The majority of obese people can have joint problems and cardiovascular limitations because of their body weight. Cardiovascular problems could include high blood pressure, high cholesterol, and even vascular issues. All of which put more pressure on the heart. These limitations are compounded by the mere fact that the heart needs to pump blood through miles of capillaries and venules of their adipose tissue. Also, careful consideration of muscle imbalances should be taken in effect. Again careful screening will tell a trainer that the individual may be prone to shoulder, knee, lower back, or hip problems that are common with obese individuals. Once the individual is properly screened and given clearance by a physician, if necessary, they can safely embark on an exercise program.

Q.) Should women lift weights if they don't want to get bulky looking? If yes, how can they lift weights and not get that bulky/masculine look?

A.) A woman getting bulky as result of weight training is a bit of myth. The average woman produces a fraction of the testosterone that men produce. Testosterone is the major hormone that separates men from women. It is also the hormone that helps men build larger amounts of muscle as compared to women. Also, building massive amounts of muscle usually involves significant changes in diet, genetics, and the mode in which you train in. Provided you are not training to build mass and the woman is not genetically predisposed to building massive amounts of muscle it is safe to say that they will not look or build muscle like a man. If you are genetically predisposed and have clear indications of higher levels of testosterone simply follow a high volume high repetition workout or circuit training and it will make it harder to build big bulky muscles.

Q.) Is it true that some people naturally lose weight faster than others? Why or why not is this the case?

A.) People are uniquely different from each other from the rate that they build muscle to the rate in which the lose weight.

Everyone's basal metabolic rate or the calories they burn at rest is different. Not to mention that some individual's genetics help them respond faster than others when it comes to losing weight. Exercise history is also important. People who have walked the path in the past more easily transition and comply more readily than an individual who has not had to comply with the necessary behavior changes for weight loss.

Q.) What precautions should seniors take into consideration, when starting a new exercise program?

A.) Senior citizens wishing to embark on an exercise regimen need to take in careful consideration of their limitations. Talk to a professional trainer or your doctor first. There are many contraindications that can arise from their age and limitations. Typically a seniors program should include exercises for posture restoration, muscle building, core strength, and conditioning. However, senior should be properly screened with a participation activity readiness questionnaire or PARQ as well as a health history questionnaire. This will inform the trainer of necessary precautions needed to avoid complications as they relate to the individuals limitations. Physical testing will also be determined by the questionnaires. Once the individual or senior has been properly assessed and screened then the trainer can properly and safely embark on a fitness program.

Q.) What are some simple things that people can do, in their day to day routine, besides working out, to see results faster?

A.) One simple thing people can do to see faster and even more results in there day to day routine, besides exercise is to eat healthy. I have heard staggering statistics such as 80-90 percent of all results associated to exercise are influenced by what they eat. This is a simple only when people see the results from exercising regularly. Changing your nutrition is not always the easiest behavior to change but it will promote the most results outside of the gym.

Q.) Is it true that it's not a good idea to do the same exercises during each workout session? Why or why not?

A.) Doing the same workout all the time is not only monotonous but it can promote muscle imbalances which can lead to injury. Also the same way our hands would callous from performing the same activity, so do our muscles. Variety is truly the spice of training. It is important to occasionally mix things up. This keeps our body guessing and constantly adapting.

Q.) How frequently should people change their workout routine?

A.) People should change their routines every 2-8 weeks depending on their goals and what they are asking their body to do. An athlete should change their program based on an event that they are trying to peak for. The average Joe should change their program to avoid repetitive motion injuries such as tendonitis and bursitis. Typically a change in their program should involve some sort of assessment or evaluation that shows progress or lack of progress. Changes should be made in order to maintain or improve progress for either the avid athlete or average Joe trying to stay in shape.

Q.) After someone has reached their fitness goals, how should their workout and nutrition plan be altered if they no longer wish to lose weight or build additional muscle?

A.) Once an individual reaches their fitness goal their program can be changed to promote maintenance, but this is not an exact science and some people need to work harder than others to maintain the current fitness level. Also the level of fitness obtained, especially if it is a high level of fitness will need more attention than an individual trying to maintain a lower level of fitness.

Q.) Is it a good idea to workout with friends or family or does that create a distraction?

A.) Working out with friends or a family member can be a distraction but in most cases it improves exercise compliance. Having a training partner can get you to the gym especially on those days that you want to go home. The fear of letting a training partner down can improve exercise compliance and facilitate results. Not to mention, that a training partner can push you harder than you would push yourself normally.

Q.) Why do people have such a hard time losing belly fat?

A.) Typically those individuals wishing to reduce belly fat are predisposed to belly fat. Every fat cell in our body from those in our cheeks to those in our belly is the same size. As we burn and lose fat our body's fat cells all shrink at the same rate. If you have noticed that your belly fat is going down. Then keep doing what you are doing. Typically those areas in which we want to see the most results with are the last to change, because they have the highest concentration of fat cells.

Q.) Is it true that it's good to have a "cheat day" where people can eat whatever they want once a week?

A.) Why is this good or bad idea? A cheat day is a great way to improve nutritional compliance. People do not typical like the idea that they will never be able to enjoy some of their favorite foods again. Having a cheat day provides not only light at the end of the tunnel, but it a reward for maintaining compliance. The same way that the body does not recognize one good nutritional day out of numerous bad days, it does not recognize one bad day out of numerous good days.

Q.) What are the best types of exercises for getting the fastest results in the shortest period of time?

A.) The exercises that produce the fastest results are exercises that impact our nervous system. The first adaption to exercise is neurological. Exercises that impact our nervous system are heavy compound movements, balance training, proprioceptive exercise, and plyometrics. It is not uncommon for a beginner to see as much as twenty percent improvement from your first workout to your second workout with heavy compound movements, balance training, proprioceptive exercise, and plyometrics.

Q.) Is it true that people with diabetes have a harder time losing weight? If so, why is this the case?

A.) People with Diabetes who exercise regularly have the most to gain from preventing some of the complications associated with diabetes as they age. Diabetes can limit the intensity in which an individual can train and what exercises the individual needs to perform in order to promote results. However because how diabetes effects the endocrine system it could make it challenging to lose weight. The pancreas and the liver are the fat burning organs of the body. Maintaining a healthy diet and properly monitoring their blood sugar levels will determine how fast and effectively the individual will lose weight.

Thank you Jeremy...

If you would like to learn more about Official Fitness Pro, their information will follow.

People can always contact me via email at jeremydancy@officialfitnesspro.com or by phone at 440-333-5365. Individuals living in the westside of Cleveland Ohio can obtain our services at any of our three locations. We offer services at the Westlake Recreation Center, Rocky River Recreation Center, or our private studio located at 19111 Detroit Rd Suite 105 Rocky River, OH 44116. For more information on our locations and services individuals can visit our website at www.officialfitnesspro.com.

Chapter (12)

SHUICHI TAKE FITNESS

"Answers provided by Shuichi Take, Owner/President"

Shuichi Take, who holds degrees in Kinesiology and Exercise Science, has over 15 years of experience in the fitness industry and has worked with hundreds of clients including professional athletes, celebrities and Fortune 500 CEO's. His Miami-based company, Shuichi Take Fitness, provides personal training services, gym management solutions and corporate wellness programs to the South Florida area.

In addition to these services, Shuichi is currently developing his website into a free national fitness resource to provide people with useful information, guidance and motivation to create healthy lifestyle habits. With relevant content such as easy-to-follow workout videos, common sense healthy meals and relatable fitness tips, Shuichi has been able to incorporate all of his experience working with individual clients over the years to create a platform that everyone can have success with, not just the rich and famous.

Shuichi's website offers a unique, interactive experience that incorporates creative social media and mobile strategies to promote visitor engagement and encourage participation. Improving your health and fitness may not be easy but with the right direction and support it doesn't have to be confusing or impossible either. The only investment Shuichi Take Fitness.com requires is a commitment to improving one's health.

Q.) What happens at the initial appointment with a personal trainer?

A.) When I first meet with a new client I like to give them some background information on me and what my fitness philosophies are. I find this to be a more effective approach then jumping right in asking them about their needs and goals as it builds a comfort level with me—an ice breaker. I also try to throw in a few jokes to make them laugh so they know I'm fun and relatable as well as give them an idea of what a workout with me would be like. Having that drill sergeant attitude or super-intense trainer image is just not my style. I don't believe you need to yell or intimidate your clients to get them to do something.

When I do get around to asking a new client about their specific fitness needs and goals I've already established some rapport with the client so they are much more candid with their responses. This ultimately allows me to get a better understanding of how a client has gotten to the state of health they are currently in and what needs to be done to assist them in improving it as well as reaching their fitness goals.

Q.) What if someone is completely out of shape? What's the safest approach for getting started?

A.) For new clients who have no exercise or workout history, baby steps is the best and only strategy. Although walking on the treadmill at 2.0mph for 5 minutes may seem easy to many people who exercise regularly, for someone who is completely out of shape it can feel like a marathon. Because their cardiovascular endurance, stamina and overall health are not the best, I focus on creating a positive experience with small successes. This builds their confidence and gives them a sense of accomplishment after every workout. This also allows me to ensure they are not overexerting themselves or risking injury by keeping the workout load light and manageable for them. By creating a workout environment that is supportive and encouraging with exercises they can accomplish can mean all the difference between a client coming back or never seeing them again.

Q.) Once someone begins working out with a personal trainer, what goes on during the sessions?

A.) Because each client has their own unique needs and goals, each workout is very different. With most of my clients, I try to avoid stagnant and repetitive routines so I mix in a variety of different fitness modalities, styles and exercises to keep things fresh and interesting. With that said, my workouts usually consist of a 5-10 minute warm-up followed by 5-10 minutes of stretching. If the client is older or has an injury I may use a longer warm-up, add more stretching or incorporate some therapy to address whatever the situation requires. If necessary, I will incorporate more stretching and additional therapy work at the end of the workout.

Because I don't believe in extended periods of rest time, I typically incorporate supersets (one exercise immediately followed by another exercise) and small circuits (a series of several exercise performed continuously). I also like to use what I call an "active break" where I have my clients do a core work or low-intensity cardio between sets to keep the heart rate up and the calories burning.

Q.) How often should someone workout with a personal trainer?

A.) Obviously, the more times a week I can work with a client the better but the reality is budget and scheduling are often limiting factors. If a client has previously worked with a trainer and/or already exercises regularly and is used to a daily routine, then 2-3 times a week is sufficient. If a client has never worked with a trainer and/or does not exercise regularly then I like to see them at least 3 times a week. The less experience a client has the more I need to see them so that we can create a habit of incorporating some form of physical activity every day.

Clients will often start working with a personal trainer and think that two workouts a week is sufficient. After a month, when they haven't seen any results, they end up blaming the trainer for not doing their job. There are 168 hours in a week so to hold your trainer responsible for the other 166 hours they are not with you is not good management of expectations or a winning strategy for success. Regardless of how many times a week I see I client, I always hold them accountable for doing their "homework" on the days I don't see them. This way they know what they need to do to get shape and have realistic expectations of what will happen if they don't fulfill their end of the agreement.

The bottom line is that in order to see results that are long-term and sustainable, you have to create a daily habit of exercising. Even if you miss a couple of days that's fine so long as you're making a conscious effort to do some form of daily physical activity. If you plan to exercise 7 days a week but only get in 4 that's still pretty good and much better than planning for 2 and only getting in one—or none!

Q.) Does it make a difference if someone just does all of their exercise over the weekend as compared to spreading it out over the week?

A.) That sounds similar to binge drinking. They say alcohol is good for you in moderation, 1-2 drinks a night promotes a healthy heart among other benefits. However, there is no health benefit to getting in your weekly alcohol quota over 2 days and the same holds true for exercising. Two really good days of exercise is not going to make up for 5 not good days. To make improvements to your health and fitness, consistent daily exercise—along with healthy eating—is the only way to achieve results. Not binging.

Q.) What is a medical release and when is it necessary?

A.) Whenever I meet with a new client for a consultation I always ask about their health history and if they have any injuries or health concerns that may affect their workout. If they give me a reason to suspect that more information is required I then proceed to dig a little deeper. If there is any concern I have for the clients well-being —as well as the well-being of my career and reputation—I then request a medical release or some form of clearance from their primary care physician. Since anything can happen during a workout, I always have clients sign a waiver of liability and indemnification agreement. This should be standard with all personal trainers.

Q.) How can a personal trainer help a client, with regard to nutrition?

A.) Most personal trainers will have enough an educational background to give clients general recommendations to improve their nutrition habits—general being something along the lines of "adding more fruits and vegetables is good for you". Personal trainers are not qualified or licensed to make specific diet or nutrition recommendations and should always refer their clients to a registered dietician or physician who is licensed in their state. They have the necessary, education, training and qualifications to assist clients with their nutrition and dietary needs. Just like a regular doctor would refer you to a specialist, a trainer should recommend their clients to a specialist when it comes to diet and nutrition.

There is a lot of debate in the in fitness community as to what is acceptable and what is not acceptable for personal trainers to recommend to their clients. My strategy has always been to share with them what I do, what the benefits are and why it works for me. Should a client want something more detailed I refer them to a dietician.

My nutrition meal plan consists of 4-5 meals a day spread out every 3-4 hours. I try to incorporate as many fruits and vegetables as I can while staying away from as much processed or refined foods as possible. I monitor my caloric intake so that it is always slightly less than my Total Daily Energy Expenditure (TDEE)—how many calories you're body burns over the course of a day from normal daily function and activity. This always keeps my body in a negative caloric balance which means I burn more calories than I take in and subsequently allows me to maintain a lean, athletic physique. Being in a negative caloric balance is the only way to burn fat and because most people want to lose weight, this is what I typically share. Should I get a client that wants to gain muscle weight I share with them my routine when I put on muscle weight; be in a positive caloric balance with most of the additional calories coming from protein. Protein supports muscle growth and muscle growth is generally why anyone would want to gain weight. Should they have any other reason to put on weight other than gaining muscle I refer them to a dietician.

Q.) What is the difference between "good fats" and "bad fats"? Which foods contain these good fats and which foods commonly contain bad fats?

A.) Unsaturated fat, the good fat which includes polyunsaturated fat and monounsaturated fats, can help lower cholesterol and reduce your risk of heart disease. Unsaturated fats are usually derived from plant and fish sources and are liquid at room temperature. A popular polyunsaturated fat is omega-3 fatty acid which is commonly found in fish oil while popular forms of monounsaturated fat are olive and canola oil. Peanuts, avocados and olives are good sources of monounsaturated fats.

Saturated fat and trans fat, the bad fat, can raise cholesterol levels, clog arteries, and increase the risk for heart disease. Saturated fats, which are solid at room temperature, are commonly found in animal products, such as meat, butter, dairy and eggs, as well as some vegetable oils such as coconut and palm oil.

There are two types of trans fats, natural trans fats and artificial trans fats. Natural trans fats are found in lean meats and low-fat dairy. Artificial trans fats, the worst of all the fats, is often used for frying or baking and is regularly used in packaged and processed foods.

Q.) Why is whole wheat bread so much better for you than white bread?

A.) Flour is made from wheat berries which are made up of 3 parts: the bran (the outer layers), the germ (the innermost area) and the endosperm (the starchy part in between). Whole wheat bread and other whole grain foods are processed to use the entire wheat berry. Wheat bread is higher in fiber which helps they digestive system and creates a feeling of fullness which can help weight control by preventing overeating. In addition to the fiber, wheat bread all has vitamins B1, B2, B6 and E, magnesium, zinc, folic acid, iron, niacin and chromium.

White bread on the other hand, has considerably less fiber, vitamins and minerals due to the way it is processed. White bread and other non-whole grain foods is processed with only the endosperm portion of the wheat berry which is mostly carbohydrates and is devoid of the nutrient and fiber rich bran and germ portion of the wheat berry.

Q.) Is it unhealthy to eat a vegetarian or vegan diet that has no meat or dairy?

A.) The main difference in a vegetarian and a vegan diet versus a regular diet is how they get their fats and protein. Vegetarians are those who do not eat any red meat (sometimes fish or chicken) but eat animal products or by-products, such as eggs and milk. Vegans, on the other hand, do not eat any meat, animal products or by-products. Vegetarians can still get some of their fats and protein from animal sources but vegans do not.

Because vegans don't have many options for sources of protein other than soy—which has its own environmental and health controversies—and nuts, some argue the vegan diet is not a healthy or sustainable for humans. Additionally, fat is essential for many normal bodily functions such as proper brain function, hormone balance and absorption of the nutrients in fruits and vegetables. Therefore, there are potential health risks with not having an adequate amount of fat in your diet which is another argument against the vegetarian and vegan diet.

With that said, I am not that proficient in either the vegetarian or vegan diet so I always advise anyone interested in either to do their due diligence and weigh the pros and cons before making a major overhaul to their nutritional habits.

Q.) Why is it better to eat more frequent, smaller meals throughout the day than less frequent larger meals?

A.) The benefit to eating more frequent, smaller meals throughout the day versus the typical 3 large meals is the effect it has on your metabolism; the rate at which your body converts food into energy when it is burned or stores it as fat when it is not burned. The idea behind smaller meals evenly spaced evenly throughout the day is that your metabolism runs at more consistent, higher level which subsequently burns more calories and stores less. Additional, by having less time between meals, you avoid hunger pains that can lead to overeating and excess calories that get stored as fat.

Q.) Why is it so important to drink water and how much water should people drink each day?

A.) The human body is made up of between 60-75% water. Drinking water and staying hydrated allows many bodily functions to run properly. Some of the bodily functions that water affects include digestion, absorption, circulation, creation of saliva, transportation of nutrients, and maintenance of body temperature. The body loses water from sweating, breathing, urine and bowel movements. When water intake is lower than output your body becomes dehydrated which can lead to serious health risks including death. Therefore, it is important to replenish water loss as soon as possible to ensure proper bodily function and health.

Q.) Is coffee bad for someone who's trying to lose weight or get in shape?

A.) Coffee contains the stimulant caffeine which has been known to increase metabolism. An increase in metabolism allows your body to burn more calories which, in turn, can help lose weight. The problem with caffeine is that your body can develop a dependency on them which results in having to constantly increase your intake to get the same effects. Therefore, I never suggest using coffee as a method of weight loss. Regular exercise to burn more calories throughout the day and healthy nutrition to take in fewer calories throughout the day is the best—and only—way to lose weight.

Q.) Every day, there seems to be a new "health food" product on the grocery store shelves. How can people tell if a food item is really healthy or not?

A.) I always advise people to get good at reading nutrition labels and ingredients of the foods they buy as well as get in the habit of counting calories so that they are more aware of what they are eating. There are many foods that may make certain claims but in reality are no better—and often times worse—than the regular version. For example, some low-fat foods may be lower in fat but higher in processed sugar.

At the end of the day, when it comes to nutrition and dieting, it's always best to consult with a registered dietician or physician to get the best professional advice. They have the background, education and expertise to answer the detailed questions that many people have about what's good and what's not good as well as what nutrition plan is best based on someone's health and fitness goals.

Thank you Shuichi…

If you would like to learn more about, Shuichi Take Fitness, their information will follow.

Shuichi Take, Owner/President

info@shuichitakefitness.com
www.shuichitakefitness.com
www.twitter.com/shuichitake
www.facebook.com/shuichitakefitness
Instagram: shuichitake

305.741.3448

1521 Alton Rd. #751
Miami Beach, FL 33139 (mailing address only)

Chapter (13)

FITNESS4LIFE TRAINING CENTER

"Answers provided by George Whitten, Owner/NASM CPT & Certified Karate Instructor"

Fitness4Life Training Center is a private training center located in Raleigh, North Carolina. We offer services that help members of our community achieve various fitness goals through a variety of group fitness programs designed to improve one's health, encourage weight loss, reduce medication for common illness, and improve daily functions like balance, coordination, flexibility, strength, agility, and stamina.

"What makes Fitness4Life different is that we have the experience to help you reach your goals and we are small enough to give you the personal attention that you need". ~George Whitten

Q.) What types of scheduling commitments are customary, when hiring a personal trainer? In other words, do people normally take things one week at a time or are they typically asked to schedule several weeks at a time with their trainer?

A.) When hiring a personal trainer most clients are expected to commit to at least eight or more sessions. Those sessions will be used based on the schedule and agreement between the client and trainer.

Q.) What should someone bring with them to a personal training session?

A.) During each personal training session make sure you have water to re-hydrate during your workout, wear comfortable clothing, and two towels. One towel will be used for personal use and the other towel can be used on equipment or the floor following other users.

Q.) What is the customary procedure, with regard to payment, if someone has to cancel an appointment with their personal trainer?

A.) When a client need to cancel a personal training session, it is customary to contact your trainer within 24 hours of your session. Such notification should be made per the agreement between the client and trainer. It is a good idea to fully understand the cancellation policy for you the client and the trainer as well. Some personal trainers will charge you for any missed session, but what happens when the trainer cannot meet you? Make sure all details are fully explained in your agreement.

Q.) Is it typical for a personal trainer to ask their clients to sign a contract? If so, what are some standard contract lengths and terms?

A.) Typically most clients do not have to sign a contract. Most clients will sign an agreement that explains the details of services provided by the trainer, the schedule for training, the cost, and other details like cancellation or renewal policies. Please note if you sign an agreement for thirty sessions and you decided to stop after twelve sessions don't expect to receive any money back unless such details are clearly stated in your agreement.

Q.) Is it better for someone to workout at home or at a gym with their personal trainer? What are the pros and cons to each?

A.) The decision to workout at home or gym really depends on the individual. If the client requires specific training and do not have the required equipment at home, then they should use the gym. When making the decision to workout at home or at the gym it really comes down to which one will you fully commit to and which one works best for your lifestyle. A good trainer can help you reach your goals at home or at a gym.

Q.) How should the diet of someone who's looking to build muscle differ from the diet of someone who's looking to lose weight?

A.) A diet for someone wanting to lose weight should have a caloric intake in excess of their daily caloric needs, and the opposite for someone wanting to lose weight. There is a lot of research stating you can eat what you want within your caloric requirement. I would not suggest you take that research literally. Considering there is about 3,500 calories in a pound, if you divide 3,500 by seven that is 500 calories per day. To grain weight you need an excess of 500 calories a day, to lose you need a deficit of 500 calories. The quality of food you consume will determine the quality of your outcome.

Q.) How long, after eating, should be people wait to workout?

A.) The time to digest food prior to a workout varies with each individual. A general rule is give yourself at least an hour and a half after eating before working out.

Q.) How should people with asthma approach their workouts?

A.) Individuals with asthma or any medical condition should first speak with their physician before starting an exercise program. Those with asthma have to be conscious of the environment; exercising in cold conditions could trigger an asthma attack, activities that are long in duration can also trigger an attack. Exercise at a level that is appropriate for you and make sure to tell your trainer you have asthma.

Q.) What are some examples of foods that people think are good for them, but they're really not, and why are these foods actually not healthy?

A.) I'm sure you've been told to stay away from processed foods. Many are unclear about what foods are considered processed. My general rule of thumb is, if it can sit on the shelves for months, even years it is processed. There are a lot of different nutrition bars, according to the labels, you are lead to believe are healthy and good for you. If you look at the ingredients you will see one of the first five ingredients is some type of sugar, and we know too much sugar in the blood raises your chances of diabetes. The other ingredients, the ones you cannot pronounce are usually chemicals the body cannot breakdown.

Q.) If someone has a favorite food that they could never give up forever, what do you suggest?

A.) Everyone has a favorite food they enjoy to eat. So, how do we focus on maintaining a healthy life and enjoy our favorites? It is alright to have those favorite temptations once in awhile. On the day you decided to have your favorite treat make sure to adjust your caloric intake accordingly. It may mean to have your favorite treat, you have to skip a meal. Most importantly, favorite treats are meant to be once in awhile, not daily!

Q.) Is it true that people can exercise their abs every day? Will this speed up their results?

A.) Abdominal muscles are like any other muscles. If you train them, they must have time to recover. If you over train muscles it takes longer to see the results you want, so train hard and get plenty of rest.

Q.)Is it true that it becomes harder to lose weight as people get older? If so, why?

A.) It becomes harder but not impossible to lose weight as you get older. Over time your metabolism slows down, the rate the body produces hormones slows down and we lose muscle mass. If you however adjust your caloric intake and stay physically active you can lose weight.

Thank you George...

If you would like to learn more about, Fitness4Life Training Center, their information will follow.

Fitness4Life Training Center is located in Raleigh, NC 27612.
Website: www.Fitness4LIfeTC.com
You can email them at info@Fitness4LIfeTC.com or call them at (919) 787-2250.
You can also like and follow them on Facebook and Twitter, www.facebook.com/fitness4lifecenter and www.twitter.com/#fitness4lifeNC.

This page intentionally left blank

Chapter (14)

RUNDLE FIT

"Answers provided by Justin Rundle, CEO"

"My name is Justin Rundle and my wife is Jessica and we are RundleFit. Jessica and I met our senior year of high school and one of our bonds has always been a mutual love for fitness. Not only do we enjoy being active, we love helping others achieve their fitness goals. After years of being successful personal trainers and strength and conditioning coaches, we felt that we could do more.

A vision developed to create a business where we could help change the health of individuals on a much larger scale. Instead of being limited to training eight clients or small groups a day, we knew we could reach thousands and provide a meaningful, healthy impact. With our population in an obesity epidemic, having an affordable, highly effective, all ability levels fitness system was a necessity.

Needless to say, we turned our dreams into a reality with our workout program called Workout Anywhere by RundleFit. Workout Anywhere is a membership site that has exclusive access to quick, effective, all ability level workouts updated every week. Membership also includes sample meal plans, recipes, challenges, motivation, coaching and a sense of community. All this is available in an easy to use mobile format for phones, tablets, computers and TV's.

Ultimately, our new weekly content and support system is designed to build healthy lifestyles, not just twelve week highlights." ~Justin Rundle

Q.) If someone needs to quickly lose a few pounds for a special occasion, what's the best way they can do this?

A.) The best way to quickly lose a few pounds for a special occasion is to increase hydration, substitute dairy and wheat with healthier alternatives and commit to total body workouts (with the H.I.I.T principle). While most consider themselves hydrated, odds are they are not. Proper hydration means consuming water and not soda, coffee, tea and alcohol. Although these drinks are okay in moderation, they do nothing for hydrating the body. Without proper hydration, one's body cannot metabolize body fat effectively or allow muscle and cellular recovery at peak performance. On top of being vital towards every health role, water is a good way to flush toxins out of the body. Toxins can create inflammation, slow one's metabolism and affect one's overall health. Which leads me to my next point?

If you want to lose weight quickly, cut out dairy and wheat. Every year the percentage of people with gluten and dairy intolerances grows. However, the reasons are becoming less of a shocker then once believed. In truth, humans are not designed to digest these products, especially when these foods contain GMO's. Hence the terms "lactose intolerant," "gluten-free," and "Wheat Belly." This can easily be explained by modern research and studies from "Forks Over Knives and other similar documentaries.

From our own experiences, weight loss has been significantly easier and easier to maintain since avoiding these foods. As well, when clients have made the same commitment to avoiding dairy and wheat, weight loss (especially fat loss) becomes more effective in a shorter amount of time. Trust me; a few years ago I wouldn't have considered myself fully lactose intolerant. In fact, I was a huge advocate for dairy products. However, I suffered from chronic digestive issues that lasted for over twenty years. It wasn't until I cut dairy that these issues went away. Every time I have tried dairy since, the problems reemerge.

Easy dairy substitutions are almond milk, coconut milk and lean proteins. Great carbohydrate substitutions for wheat are quinoa, sweet potatoes and fruit (in moderation).

To compliment all of these substitutions and to burn the maximum amount of body fat in the shortest amount of time, give total body workouts with the principle of High Intensity Interval Training a try. This is also known as metabolic conditioning and is the perfect regimen for building lean muscle while incinerating fat. Workouts can range from sprints, with rest periods. Total body strength training circuits with limited rest periods and just about any combination of strength, conditioning, core and plyometric training one can think of. As long the rest periods are controlled and moderated workouts can be completed in as little as 20 minutes or less.

Best thing about this style, if a trainer really knows what they are doing; they can adapt this program to suit all ability levels. H.I.I.T may sound scary, but it is truly scalable for all ability levels as long as the trainer and client have great communication, heart rate zones are established and the trainer understands the client's fitness level and capabilities.

Q.) Does a person have to check with their doctor before beginning a workout program with a personal trainer?

A.) A person should always check with their doctor before beginning a workout program with a personal trainer. Ultimately, the client will use their own discretion, but as a trainer, you should always make it clear the client or future client that they should have a physical beforehand.

Most doctors will fully support a good fitness and nutrition program, as it is the easiest and most practical investment one can make in their own health. However, it is important for the trainer to know of any health or fitness limitations of the client.

Q.) What types of shoes should people wear when working out?

A.) The best shoes for an overall fitness program are cross-trainers. Having a shoe that's versatile and supportive for most activities is crucial to total body fitness programs. Running shoes are great for running, but they are designed for lateral support or constructed for weight training.

Q.) In addition to working out, what are some of the most beneficial activities to participate in and why are these activities so beneficial/healthy?

A.) The elements that are the true game changers to a fitness program are actually nutrition, rest and a supportive environment. Nutrition is literally 80% of a determining factor for any fitness goal. For most people, it is almost impossible to outwork their diet. People feel as though they just put themselves through a grueling workout that they can eat and drink whatever they feel like. In reality, most efficient workouts burn around 300-600 calories during the workout. In one sitting with the typical American diet, one can ingest between 800-2,000 calories. The math doesn't add up towards weight loss. I'm not solely a proponent on calories in versus calories out. There are certainly other variables that go into one's daily calorie expenditure. However, until whole and organic foods become mainstream, those statistics are going to around for a while.

Rest is the body's prime time to recover, regrow and recharge. The body utilizes this with well-timed rest days and healthy sleep patterns. In fact, the body burns calories in its deep R.E.M sleep cycle to rebuild muscle fiber, promote cellular repair and recharge. Some wonder why they are not losing weight when their nutrition and fitness are on point, but their sleep pattern is a wreck. Once this missing link is corrected, the whole process runs smoothly.

A supportive, encouraging environment can be crucial to a successful transition into a healthy lifestyle. Generally, our clients who made a commitment to their new and improved health with their spouse, friend or peer group are more likely to obtain their fitness goals then the lone wolfs. This is not always so, but more often then not, a team is stronger then the individual. This also curbs stress (cortisol), which can be detrimental to a body transformation.

Q.) Why do people say, "Breakfast is the most important meal of the day"? Is there any truth in this?

A.) Breakfast is the most important meal of the day because it jump-starts the metabolism out of the fast by breaking the fast of the night's slumber. As well, breakfast regulates ones insulin. This in turn creates a more energetic, focused you for the rest of the day. If one skips this meal, they are more likely to binge during the later hours on sugary, high carb and high calorie snacks. This can in turn lead to Type 2 Diabetes according to Harvard School of Public Health.

Q.) What are the best foods that people should eat to gain energy and why are these foods so important?

A.) For natural energy, add more raw fresh fruits and vegetables into your diet. Eat them raw, or juice them to extract all the phytonutrients, live enzymes and antioxidants. The results are amazing for one's health, energy and mental focus. Much better then caffeine.

Q.) Is it better to lift weights with free weights or with weight machines? Why is one better than the other?

A.) Free weights are far better than machines because of the "free" aspect. One has to be in total control and focused when using free weights. That said, more muscle groups, stabilizer muscles and one's core become a factor when going free.

Machines are guided and meant for isolating a muscle, or muscle group. However, due to the guided nature, less muscle groups are involved with supporting the exercise. Machines are great for rehabilitation or completely isolating a muscle, but for more of a caloric burn and overall body strength training, free weights are the prime choice.

Q.) Is it true that eating too many vegetables will make most people gain water weight?

A.) The main contributor to water retention is sodium and toxins. If one is increasing their vegetables without reducing their sodium intake, then odds are they will retain water. As well, if one is not decreasing the overly processed or synthetic foods in their daily diet, it is possible to have an inflammatory response. The best way to combat inflammation and water retention is to drink more water and have plenty of vegetables and fruits. Antioxidants from fruits and veggies are crucial for warding off free radicals that come from inflammation.

Q.) How can someone do resistance training if they don't own weights or belong to a gym?

A.) It's actually not necessary to belong to a gym to obtain optimal results when it comes to resistance training. As well, a gym can be a major distraction due to social circles, added commute time and sharing or waiting on equipment. If someone wants a quick and effective home workout, all they need is a good attitude and their own body. In fact, gymnasts rarely touch a weight. The body weight movements they use and they way they can manipulate their own bodies takes an incredible amount of strength and core control. With the ability to manipulate ones body, the endless array of non-equipment core training exercises, plyometric training and conditioning drills, one can have the strongest and fittest physique of their life without weights or a gym. People who commit to home workouts are focused on their goal and know that time is of the essence. This is our specialty.

Q.) Do people really lose muscle as they get older? If so, how much muscle do they lose on average, and can anything be done to slow down this process?

A.) I used to believe that people lose muscle as they get older, due to naturally decreasing HGH and hormone levels. However, my beliefs have shifted. Over the years, my wife and I have worked with a number of clients who initially believed this. Their friends and peers already believed this misconception, so their activity level and strength training routine fit accordingly. That means that for whatever reason, the people who fall into this category all seem to adopt a light resistance and moderate conditioning training program along with a typical American diet. This is the perfect formula to lose muscle gradually. Our clients in the aging category have all experienced overall increases in strength and lean muscle. As well, the perfect compliment to our beliefs is the true life account of Dr. Jeffry S. Life titled, "The Life Plan: How Any Man Can Achieve Lasting Health, Great Sex, and a Stronger, Leaner Body."

Q.) How can someone figure out how many calories they should be eating each day?

A.) The Basal Metabolic Rate formula is the standard for determining the energy expenditure at rest. With it, one can compare energy in to energy out for a more precise caloric allowance. Generally for a female with a weight loss goal, the range will be 1,200 to 1,600 calories a day. For males, 2,200 to 2,800. An easier way to use this formula is with apps like Livestrong's My Plate and My Fitness Pal to have all this calculated for you.

The most precise tool for keeping track of one's daily calorie allowance is the Body Media Fit Link Armband as seen on the Biggest Loser. This instrument takes real time calculations by reading one's heat and energy expenditure along with heart rate.

Q.) Is it true that muscle will turn to fat if someone stops working out?

A.) This is a huge misconception. Muscle tissue cannot physically turn into fatty tissue. However, the reason this is presumed is because a lack of activity causes muscle atrophy and promotes more body fat storage. If one's lean muscle tissue is not using calories to function and grow, but the body is used to a certain level of activity, then it's more likely to store this energy (fat cells equal stored energy).

Q.) What is "body fat percentage"? How does this differ from "body mass index"?

A.) Body fat percentage is a figure used to determine how much of one's body non-lean tissue (body fat) is. One's overall body composition consists of water, muscle, body fat and skeletal percentages.

Body Mass Index is a number calculated from one's height and weight to determine what weight one should be at for health screening purposes. However, it doesn't take into account one's body type. It's a standard that is extremely outdated.

Q.) What can thin people do to build muscle?

A.) The best way for thin people to build muscle is by creating a calorie surplus of whole, organic, nutrient dense proteins, carbohydrates and fats while using a hypertrophy style strength-training program. It doesn't do a skinny person any good to fill their body up with a bunch of sludge just to promote lean muscle growth. Instead, give the body a surplus of nutrient dense food. This will promote strength and muscle gains with a mass building (hypertrophy) program.

Thank you Justin...

If you would like to learn more about, Rundle Fit, their information will follow.

Contact Justin or Jessica Rundle at www.workoutanywhere.net, for more assistance with your health, fitness and nutrition goals.

This page intentionally left blank

Chapter (15)

FITNESS BY PATTY

*"Answers provided by Patty Soud,
Certified Personal Trainer"*

Fitness By Patty is dedicated to helping people discover their 'whole-body fitness' by leading an organically healthy lifestyle, eating clean, and exercising daily. She believes the healthier you are, the more you can do, and the better you can do it. Fitness By Patty teaches people that proper nutrition, regular exercise, and quality sleep are the most important things you can do for your body, and that together, these components deliver to you the most natural form of medicine. Fitness By Patty takes a very personal and holistic approach to creating personal exercise routines combined with balanced, whole-foods nutrition in respect to one's body. Fitness By Patty offers In-Home Personal Training (individuals, partners, small groups), Range Of Motion Stretch Therapy, Aquatic Fitness, and Corporate Wellness Fitness & Nutrition Programs.

Q.) What exactly does a personal trainer do?

A.) Before all else, a personal trainer listens to her client's desires, needs, and goals. Then, she formulates a safe and healthy plan to help take that client from their starting line, and carefully progresses them into exercises and custom-designed training phases that are suitable to their level of fitness, with a side of creativity and functionality as it relates to their sport, activity or lifestyle.

Q.) If someone hasn't worked out in years, how should they get started in the safest way possible?

A.) It is preferred, that if someone has not worked out in years, to have a physical done by their primary doctor, to ensure all systems are on 'go'. Once clearance for physical fitness/workout routine is granted, the safest way to begin is to simply start moving, ie: walking (if able/accessible). The best way to ensure you are going to benefit from your exercises and efforts toward workouts is to meet with a reputable, trusted, and certified personal trainer. She can learn about your health history, any potential injuries or medical conditions that may need exercise modifications, and begin to develop a safe and enjoyable routine that you can do a few times a week. Slow and steady is the name of the game when it comes to getting back into the swing of things. It's better to know you're starting back the right way, rather than to try an old workout trick you may have seen your gym buddies doing years ago because it looked cool (which may actually be harmful to certain parts of your body).

Q.) Can couples or groups of people workout with a personal trainer at the same time?

A.) Absolutely. When couples or groups of people workout with the personal trainer, everyone wins! The clients get a discounted rate for personal training, as well as an extra motivation (from other participants enduring the same hard work) and the trainer gets paid a little more for her time, and is able to help more people become fit and healthy at the same time.

Q.) Is it safe to workout first thing in the morning, on an empty stomach?

A.) Yes it is safe, as long as you have a little something of substance still in your stomach from the night before and are hydrated, as well as plan to eat post-workout. There are 2 different types of people; Those who workout in the mornings before starting their day, and those who workout at the end of the day. People have different body types, sleep habits, energy levels, etc. So for some people, working out first thing in the morning is what helps to wake them up, put them in a good mood, and be productive with a clear mind. On the other hand, there are also people who feel they perform better after they've been up for hours, (working, etc.) have a little something in their stomach a couple hours before the workout. Because they can de-stress from their busy day with a workout, and it also helps them sleep better when they exercise in the evenings.

Q.) Do personal trainers usually have insurance?

A.) Yes, personal trainers (if they're smart) usually have insurance. No matter how good they are, how long they've been training, etc., you NEVER know what could happen. Personal trainers should be viewed as someone you can trust to know what to do with your body, and how hard to push your limits (or not push too far), but no matter what - insurance is a must.

Q.) How can people, with very busy work schedules and family commitments, fit working out into their schedule?

A.) The way busy people fit working out into their schedules typically happens best if it is done as an appointment time, just like any other important task. Scheduling time for workouts should not feel like a chore, but viewed more as a necessary daily habit like brushing your teeth and eating breakfast. Family commitments could be either an excuse not to workout, or an opportunity to include them in the exercise as well. Working out doesn't always mean you have to go to the gym, be away for an hour or more and miss out on important work and family commitments. There are tons of ways to get a good workout in by small bouts of time (intervals) or by combining more full body exercises into the same routine if you're looking to workout in a time-constricted window.

Q.) How many grams of fat should people consume each day, if they want to lose weight?

A.) Depending on the daily caloric goal of the individual looking to lose weight, generally speaking, you should take about 20-30% of your daily caloric needs, and then divide that number by 9, which accounts for the calories from fat grams. Best to also choose quality sources of fat to make up the recommended amounts per day ie: unsalted nuts, avocado, extra virgin olive oil, etc.

Q.) What are some of the most common myths about building muscle?

A.) Some of the most common myths about building muscle are that you need to consume more protein. ACSM recommends that "endurance and strength-trained athletes" have between 1.2 and 1.7 g/kg (.5 - .8 grams per pound) of protein for the best performance and health. The best way to calculate your protein needs is:

1. Take your weight in pounds, divided by 2.2 = your weight in kg.

2. Take your weight in kg x 0.8 - 1.8gm/kg = protein gm.

(Use the lower number if you are in good health and sedentary, and use a higher number if you are pregnant, recovering from illness, or participating in intense endurance or weight training.)

Q.) Do people need exercise equipment to get in shape?

A.) It is not a necessity for people to have equipment to get in shape. Body weight training is very effective, and as long as you have a mix of different exercises that can work all of the major muscle groups, you will end up feeling the results from your own body weight as your equipment. If you wanted a cheap investment for something extra to challenge you to the next level in your training, you could use simple resistant bands, or even some 1/2 to 1 gallon jugs to serve as your 'free weights'.

Q.) What is a healthy amount of weight to lose each week? Why is it a bad idea to lose more weight than this each week?

A.) It is safe to lose 1-2 lbs of weight per week. Your body responds better when change happens gradually and safely (balanced nutrition and regular daily exercise). Although from a beginner's stand point, you may begin your exercise and healthy eating routine, and lose up to 5 lbs in a week because of the shock to your body. However, this much weight loss per week will not be a healthy amount to continue losing. Constantly trying to lose more than 1-2 lbs per week over time will be more detrimental to your health, as you could be stripping more nutrition from your body than you realize, and your organs depend on that nutritional balance, caloric intake versus caloric expenditure.

Q.) If someone belongs to a gym, how can they get their personal trainer into the gym they're a member of?

A.) Typically, it is frowned upon to bring your (non-gym employed) trainer into your gym (where there are other personal trainers for hire, on staff). However, people still do it all the time, for different reasons. If you want to 'make nice' with the gym you are a member of, just let one of the managers know that you have already hired a trainer and prefer not to use one of theirs (maybe you have a special health/medical condition). They can refuse your request, or they may just have you pay an extra fee and call them a guest. But to be civil, hopefully your trainer won't try to attract too much attention to themselves by "motivating" you too loudly, or taking up floor space by doing "new exercises". Respect the gym, respect it's members, and respect your trainer (so she doesn't feel awkward/looked down upon in a place where she is not even employed).

Q.) There seems to be a lot of talk about these "cleansing diets", where people just drink lemon juice with cayenne pepper and some sort of syrup for 30 or more days. Is this safe and/or healthy? Why or why not?

A.) This kind of "diet" is not healthy, and it is definitely not safe because our bodies are made to intake proper amounts of macro-nutrients on a daily basis, in moderation. There are times when our bodies can safely cleanse in a couple of days (2-3) on a fruit and vegetable diet, but 30 or more days is just absurd. Those types of diets never last, and by the end of the 30 or more days, your body will go into reverse mode and can develop a mess of gastrointestinal problems at the least, which you will end up paying for in the long run, for trying to fix your body of the damage done.

Q.) Is weight lifting a good idea for people who have high blood pressure?

A.) Strength training is still a good way for people who have high blood pressure to help lower their blood numbers, especially if it is light to moderate weights with higher repetitions, and proper breathing techniques, as well as intermittent rest periods. Another reason to consult with your physician before starting a workout routine, then hiring a trusted, certified and experienced personal trainer.

Q.) Is it dangerous to take supplements?

Depending on the supplements you want to take, if they are more than what your doctor recommends because of a low amount of a certain vitamin or mineral, they are dangerous. You are better off eating a healthy balanced whole-foods, more plant-based diet than trying to take a special supplement to aid in weight/fat loss, or help boost your energy with chemicals that aren't found in real foods.

Thank you Patty...

If you would like to learn more about Fitness By Patty, their information will follow.

Patty Soud operates Fitness by Patty and is located in Atlantic Beach, Florida.
Phone number: 904.699.2262.
Email: Patty@FitnessByPatty.com.
Website: www.FitnessByPatty.com
Blog: www.FitnessByPatty.com/blog
Fitness By Patty is also on Pinterest, Facebook, Twitter, Yelp, Google Plus, and Linked In.

This page intentionally left blank

CONCLUSION

Congratulations on making it to the end of this book! We hope that you realize and appreciate the immense level of real world knowledge that you've just acquired. The one thing you may be feeling, at this point, is a bit of "information overload", due to the many tips, pieces of advice, and strategies that are jammed into this book. If you are feeling a bit overwhelmed from everything you've just learned, allow us to offer you one final piece of advice: Take a day to let your brain absorb all of the information you just learned. As they say: "Sleep on it". If you attempt to try and remember and implement everything you just learned, your efforts may tend to be scattered and a bit unorganized. Instead, take a day off from the information. If you do this, you're likely to find that you develop a sense of clarity and a better perspective on the information.

Once you've taken a day to allow yourself to re-focus in this way, we encourage you to slowly go back through the book, writing

down the actionable information that you intend to implement. Simply reading and understanding the information is not enough. By writing down the information that you plan on implementing, it will allow you to put a clear plan of action into place for yourself.

As you go through the information, don't worry about the order in which you write things down. The first thing to do is to just get the information down on paper. There are many great strategies and tips within this book, but the goal here is for you to extract the exact advice that you will be taking action on. Don't worry if you are unsure about whether or not you will be taking immediate action on certain advice. Just write down everything that you may possibly take action on.

Once you've compiled this list of action steps and "maybe action steps", begin to prioritize this list. In other words, re-write the list with the actions that you know you're going to take at the top of the list and the action items that you may not take action on towards the bottom of the list. By organizing your list in this way, you will be able to build a practical, useable to-do list, from the information you learned in this book. Once you've done this, you will be in an excellent position to start taking focused steps, with clarity and purpose.

As we mentioned at the beginning of this book, most peddlers or fitness products and information hope that you keep buying their stuff. In keeping with the rebellious nature of this book, we encourage you to stop buying more fitness stuff and start implementing what you just learned in this book! Just as we have shared interviews with real world experts who actually do what they talk about in this book, it is our hope that you, as the reader, will take real world action on the information you've learned here.

Wishing you all the best in your action-taking, fitness and nutrition endeavors!